contents

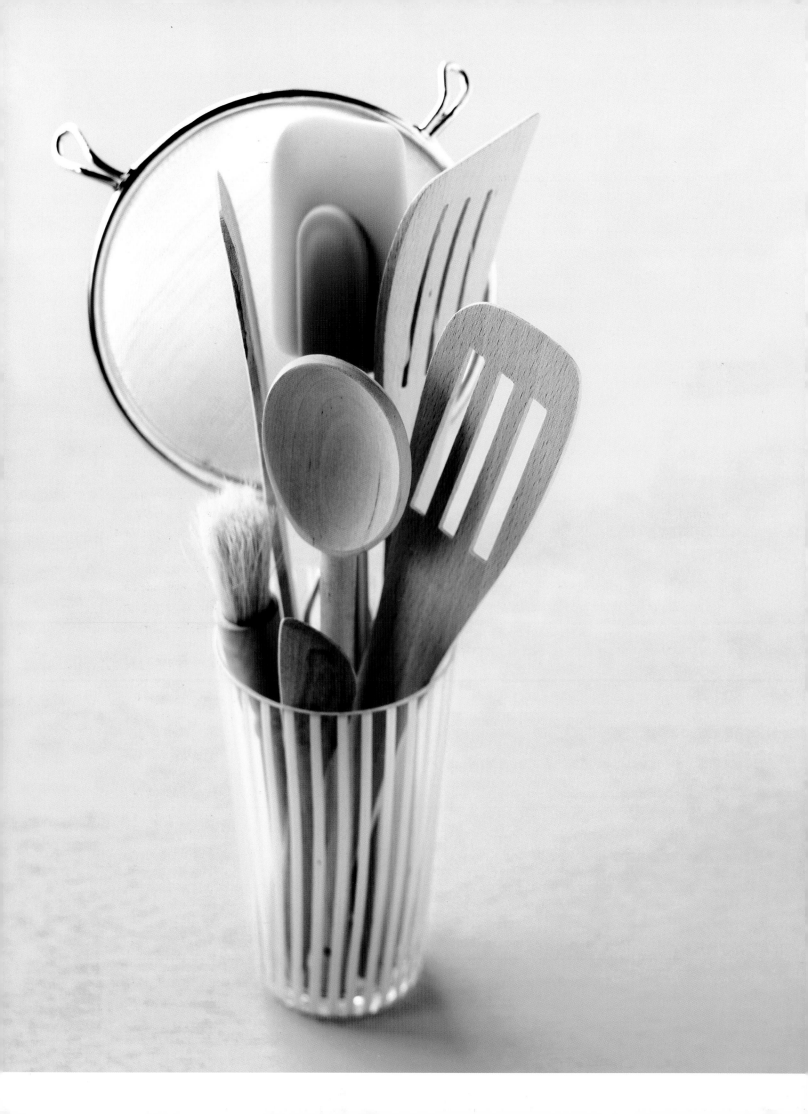

introduction

Diabetes is a complex metabolic disease that affects the whole body. Although there are different types of diabetes, they all result in too much sugar being present in the bloodstream. There is currently no cure for the disease, but there are steps you can take to reduce your risk of developing diabetes or to control the condition once you have it.

During the last two decades, the number of people being diagnosed with diabetes has rapidly increased in all affluent societies around the world. Almost ten per cent of people living in western countries have diabetes. Having excess body fat and being inactive increases your risk of developing type 2 diabetes, particularly if you have a family history of diabetes.

what is diabetes?

Diabetes is a condition where the amount of sugar (glucose) in the blood is excessively high. This is because the body is either not producing enough insulin or it is not reacting to it properly.

After a person consumes food or drink that contains carbohydrate (sugar or starch), the level of glucose sugar in their bloodstream rises as the carbohydrate is digested into glucose and absorbed into the blood. In people without diabetes, the rise in the blood's glucose level stimulates the pancreas to release the hormone insulin, which enables the body's cells to absorb the glucose from the blood to use as energy, causing the blood's glucose level to fall back to normal. In people with diabetes, the pancreas doesn't make sufficient insulin or their cells don't respond to it properly, so glucose is not effectively taken up from the bloodstream.

Consequently, after a person with untreated diabetes eats a meal, their blood glucose rises to a higher level and remains higher than normal for a longer time. The hormone insulin also helps the body to absorb digested fats and proteins from the bloodstream. Over time, the high blood glucose and fat levels in people with poorly controlled diabetes can damage their eyes, nerves and blood vessels, and also increases the risk of developing heart disease, kidney and circulatory problems. Early diagnosis and treatment of diabetes are essential for avoiding these serious health problems.

types of diabetes

There are three main types of diabetes: type 1 diabetes; type 2 diabetes; and gestational diabetes.

type 1 diabetes

Type 1 diabetes, also known as insulin-dependent diabetes, is the most serious but least common type of diabetes. In the past it has been referred to as juvenile-onset diabetes because it mostly arises during childhood. However, it can also occur in adults, typically under 30 years of age. Type 1 diabetes usually results from an autoimmune disease (not from eating too much sugar). The body's immune system starts destroying the pancreas, and eventually the pancreas stops producing sufficient (if any) insulin. It is thought that exposure to a certain chemical or virus may trigger the autoimmune reaction in some genetically susceptible people.

The autoimmune process that damages the pancreas can develop quickly or over several years. However, the symptoms of type 1 diabetes usually appear quite abruptly and quickly get worse. Symptoms include excessive thirst and frequent urination (the kidneys are working harder to try to flush out the excess glucose from the bloodstream); unintentional weight loss (generally rapid in children and slower in adults); extreme fatigue; blurred vision; abdominal cramps; nausea; and vomiting.

People who have type 1 diabetes require daily insulin injections to stay alive. These injections must be balanced with their food intake, exercise, health, and stress levels, and be guided by regular blood glucose measurements.

type 2 diabetes

Type 2 diabetes, which is also known as non-insulin dependent or adult-onset diabetes, is the most common type of diabetes. It usually occurs in adults over 30 years of age, but has recently started increasing in children and teenagers, most of whom are overweight, relatively inactive and have a family history of diabetes. Type 2 diabetes occurs when the body is no longer responding properly to insulin (insulin resistance) and/or the pancreas is no longer producing enough insulin. When a person becomes insulin resistant, their pancreas tries to compensate by producing more insulin than normal whenever the blood's glucose level rises. It is thought that the increased rate of insulin production may eventually exhaust the pancreas, particularly if the person's insulin resistance continues to get worse. Unless their blood glucose level is very high, people with type 2 diabetes may not have any noticeable symptoms and may not be aware that they have the condition. However, possible symptoms include excessive thirst; frequent urination; blurred vision; thrush; increased susceptibility to infections (in the gums, skin and feet); and weight loss.

Different people with type 2 diabetes have different genetic and metabolic factors and will be at varying stages of the disease when diagnosed, so there is no one ideal diet or medical therapy that will suit all people with type 2 diabetes. Individualised treatment is required. Some people can successfully manage their condition by controlling their weight with healthy eating and regular exercise. Other people require medication, such as tablets that reduce the insulin resistance, as well as lifestyle changes to keep their blood sugar level under control. Some people with type 2 diabetes eventually require daily insulin injections in order to gain sufficient control of their blood sugar level.

gestational diabetes

Gestational diabetes (GD) is a form of diabetes (usually temporary) that develops in about three per cent of pregnant women. It occurs when the mother cannot produce all of the insulin required for her body's increased needs during pregnancy. GD usually appears in the second or third trimester and disappears once the pregnancy is over. It is usually detected during a routine blood test at 24 to 28 weeks and is generally treated with healthy eating alone, although in some cases the mother needs hospitalisation and insulin therapy.

GD should not be taken lightly, because if left untreated it can result in miscarriage, stillbirth, a difficult delivery, and health problems in the infant. GD significantly increases both the mother's and child's risk of developing type 2 diabetes later in life, but the risk can be reduced in both mother and child with a healthy diet and regular physical activity.

pre-diabetes

There is a pre-diabetic condition where the blood glucose level is higher than normal but not yet in the diabetic range. This is present when a person has:

◆ **impaired fasting glucose** – when their blood sugar level is higher than normal after a period of fasting (such as on waking in the morning); or
◆ **impaired glucose tolerance** – when their blood sugar level rises to a higher level than normal after eating due to greater insulin resistance.

Pre-diabetes significantly increases the risk of developing type 2 diabetes if left untreated. However, you can completely reverse pre-diabetes or stop it progressing to diabetes simply by improving your lifestyle. Recent large-scale research studies have shown that people with impaired glucose tolerance

risk factors for type 2 diabetes

◆ You are more than 45 years old with high blood pressure and excess body fat, and you do little physical activity or you have a family history of diabetes.
◆ You are more than 35 years old and of Asian, Polynesian, Aboriginal, Torres Strait Islander, Southern European, Hispanic or Indian descent.
◆ You are more than 55 years old.
◆ You have a parent or sibling with diabetes.
◆ You have had a heart attack or stroke or you have heart disease.

◆ You have gestational diabetes or your baby weighed more than 4 kg at birth.
◆ You have polycystic ovary syndrome (PCOS).
◆ You are overweight and are apple-shaped rather than pear-shaped (you store more fat on your upper body than on your hips and thighs).
◆ You have pre-diabetes.
◆ You have high blood pressure and/or high blood cholesterol and/or triglycerides.

can avoid developing type 2 diabetes simply by controlling their body weight (losing at least five per cent of excess body weight); reducing their fat intake; increasing their fibre intake; and getting at least 30 minutes of moderate exercise each day. These simple lifestyle improvements resulted in greater protection against diabetes than the standard medication that is prescribed to treat pre-diabetes.

As little as 40 minutes a day of moderate physical activity, such as brisk walking, coupled with some weight loss, not only makes you look and feel better, but significantly improves your overall health and greatly reduces your risk of developing diabetes and other serious health problems.

managing your diabetes

The main treatment goal for any type of diabetes is to try to keep your blood glucose level within the normal range (or as close as possible to the upper limit of the range), in order to avoid developing the long-term health problems associated with diabetes, such as heart disease, kidney failure and blindness. Healthy eating, regular physical activity and weight control all reduce the amount of insulin your body needs and are the key tools for controlling your blood sugar, cholesterol and blood pressure levels. Some people may also need certain medication along with a healthy lifestyle to help them control their diabetes. It is important to remember that medication should not take the place of a healthy lifestyle — it should be used together with healthy eating and regular exercise for maximum effect.

tips for managing diabetes

- Eat a healthy low-GI diet.
- Maintain a healthy weight.
- Get regular physical activity.
- Reduce your stress levels.
- Take any medication prescribed for you.
- Don't smoke.
- Drink alcohol in moderation, if at all.
- Learn how to measure your blood glucose level and interpret the results.
- See your doctor and other health professionals on a regular basis.

healthy eating for diabetes

Diabetes is a metabolic problem and is greatly affected by the quantity and quality of food a person chooses to eat. Advances in scientific research in the last 30 years have greatly improved the dietary recommendations for people with diabetes, which are now less strict than they used to be.

The 'healthy diet pyramid' model applies to people with and without diabetes, because people living in western countries generally have a high risk of developing nutrition-related diseases, such as diabetes and heart disease. Most of the food that you eat should be vegetables, fruit, legumes and wholegrain cereal products that have a low Glycemic Index (GI), accompanied by moderate amounts of lean protein-rich foods (lower-fat dairy products and alternatives, lean meats and poultry, eggs, fish and seafood). Small quantities of fat from healthy foods can also be included in the daily diet, such as nuts, seeds, avocados, olives and olive oil. A variety of healthy foods should be eaten each day, including different coloured fruit and vegetables. Alcohol and 'junk' foods should not be consumed on a regular basis. Aim to make your diet as natural as possible.

Different people need different amounts of food, and many people with type 2 diabetes would benefit from losing some weight. It is very useful to consult a dietitian, who can develop a meal plan that suits your needs, particularly if you are newly diagnosed or you also have another health problem such as a food allergy. You may need to see a dietitian and a diabetes educator every week or two for the first few months after you have been diagnosed in order to learn how to control and measure your blood sugar level at home. After that, it's still worth seeing a dietitian at least every 6 to 12 months to fine-tune your diet.

the glycemic index

In the past, it was assumed that sugars (previously called simple carbohydrates) contained in foods and drinks would be more quickly digested than starches (complex carbohydrates) and would cause a greater rise in blood glucose. This assumption was based on the fact that sugars are smaller molecules than starches. However, when scientists actually measured the blood glucose (glycemic) responses produced by different foods, they found that this assumption wasn't correct. In fact, the amount of sugar or starch in a food is not a good indication of its blood glucose effect, but the type of sugar or starch is.

There are a number of different types of sugars and starches in foods, which vary in their chemical composition and the rate at which they are digested and absorbed. Foods and drinks that contain rapidly digested carbohydrate produce a relatively high blood glucose response, whereas foods and drinks that contain slowly digested carbohydrate produce a lower blood glucose response (see graph below). Certain processing and cooking methods increase the digestibility of carbohydrates in food by changing the chemical structure of the carbohydrate or breaking it down into smaller pieces. The more processed a food is, the easier it is to digest and the higher it sends your blood glucose level. For example, white bread has a higher GI than coarse wholegrain bread, and mashing or pureeing starchy foods, such as potatoes, increases their GI.

In the 1980s, scientists developed the Glycemic Index (GI) method to measure the extent to which different carbohydrate-rich foods increase the blood's glucose level after being eaten. The GI method ranks equal-carbohydrate portions of different carbohydrate-containing foods and drinks according to the blood glucose response they produce after they are eaten (equal-carbohydrate portions of foods are used, because carbohydrate causes the blood's glucose level to rise). Therefore, only foods and drinks that have significant amounts of carbohydrate can have a GI value.

Foods and drinks with a high GI value (70 or more) contain carbohydrate that is rapidly digested and absorbed and produces a fast and large rise in blood glucose. Low-GI (55 or less) foods and drinks contain carbohydrate that is digested and absorbed at a relatively slow rate (or they contain predominantly fructose or lactose sugar). Medium-GI (56 to 69) foods produce intermediate blood glucose responses.

Traditionally, people with diabetes were advised to eat specific amounts of carbohydrate at certain times of the day. They were given a carbohydrate exchange list so they could select their target carbohydrate amount from different foods. This system has now been replaced with the GI system in many countries, where people with diabetes or pre-diabetes are advised to choose low-GI carbohydrate-rich foods as part of a balanced diet. However, a low-GI diet is not only relevant for people with diabetes. It offers health benefits for everyone. Scientific research shows that a healthy low-GI diet and regular exercise will lower your risk of developing diabetes and other health problems.

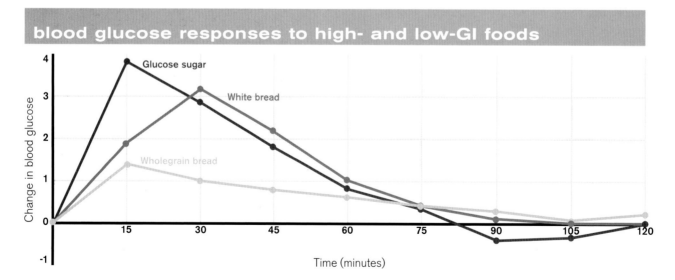

blood glucose responses to high- and low-GI foods

This graph shows typical blood glucose responses in a healthy person after they have eaten an equal-carbohydrate portion of glucose sugar, white bread and wholegrain bread (each food was eaten on a separate day). The person started eating at 0 minutes and finished after 10 minutes and their blood sugar level was measured every 15 minutes for the next 2 hours. Glucose sugar (GI = 100) is rapidly absorbed into the bloodstream, causing a fast and large rise in blood glucose. High-GI white bread contains rapidly digested starch. Low-GI wholegrain bread contains more slowly digested starch.

a guide for switching from high-GI foods to low-GI foods

higher-GI foods	lower-GI foods
bakery food	
◆ white bread, buns, bagels, Lebanese bread	◆ dense wholegrain bread, wholegrain English muffins
◆ light wholemeal or rye bread	◆ dense bread made from stone-ground flour
◆ crumpets, scones, white English muffins	◆ pumpernickel bread
◆ pancakes, pikelets, waffles	◆ sourdough bread
◆ croissants	◆ stone-ground pita bread
◆ lower-fat biscuits, crackers and crispbreads	◆ biscuits with dried fruit, oats and/or whole grains
◆ puffed corn cakes, puffed rice cakes, rice crackers	◆ bakery goods made with stone-ground flour and a
◆ bakery goods made with fine white flour and sugar	low-calorie sweetener suitable for baking
grains & legumes	
◆ most long- and short-grain rices (white and brown),	◆ basmati rice, Doongara rice, koshikari rice, wild rice
including arborio risotto rice, broken rice, glutinous rice,	◆ barley, buckwheat, bulgur wheat, quinoa
instant rice, jasmine rice	◆ all types of legumes (for example chickpeas, kidney beans,
◆ couscous, millet, polenta (cornmeal), puffed amaranth	lentils, soybeans, split peas)
◆ broad beans	
pasta & noodles	
◆ gluten-free corn pasta, gluten-free rice pasta	◆ durum wheat pasta
◆ gnocchi	◆ meat-filled ravioli or tortellini
◆ dried rice noodles, udon noodles	◆ dried buckwheat soba noodles, fresh rice noodles,
◆ low-fat instant noodles	mung bean (glass) noodles
starchy vegetables	
◆ beetroot, parsnips, potatoes, pumpkin, swedes	◆ carrots, cassava, corn, green peas, orange sweet potato, yam
breakfast cereals	
◆ processed breakfast cereals based on puffed or	◆ natural muesli without flaked or puffed grains
flaked grains	◆ porridge made from wholegrain rolled oats or rolled barley
◆ bran flakes, cornflakes, puffed rice, puffed wheat,	◆ semolina
wheat biscuits (plain)	◆ oat bran, rice bran
fruit	
◆ bananas (very ripe), breadfruit, dark cherries, pawpaw,	◆ apples, bananas (not overripe), berries, citrus fruit, custard
pineapple, rockmelon, watermelon	apples, grapes, kiwifruit, mangoes, nectarines, peaches,
◆ raisins, dried dates	pears, plums, tomatoes
◆ canned lychees in syrup	◆ dried apples, dried apricots, dried pears, prunes
dairy & alternatives	
◆ rice milk	◆ cow's milk, soy milk
◆ sweetened condensed milk	◆ most ice creams
◆ some highly sweetened ice creams and ice cream-	◆ custard
like desserts	◆ yoghurt, fromage frais

Some low-GI foods, such as chocolate and potato chips, are low GI because of their high fat content (the large amount of fat slows down the rate of carbohydrate digestion). These types of low-GI foods are not recommended for everyday eating due to their high fat content.

Just because a food has a low GI value doesn't mean it is necessarily a good choice for people with diabetes. If the food isn't a fruit, vegetable, wholegrain cereal product or low-fat dairy product (or alternative), then it's not a low-GI food that should be eaten on a regular basis.

the benefits of a low-GI diet

Many scientific research studies have shown that a low-GI, lower-fat diet improves blood glucose control, lowers high blood cholesterol, and can reduce weight gain and the risk of heart disease in people with diabetes or pre-diabetes. Simply replacing the high-GI foods in your diet with lower-GI alternatives will improve your blood glucose control and reduce your body's need for insulin.

Basing your diet on low-GI foods is very helpful for weight control. Less processed low-GI foods (such as traditional wholegrain rolled oats and wholegrain bread) are generally more filling than their high-GI counterparts (such as instant oats and white bread) because they are more difficult to chew and swallow and take longer to digest.

Some people with type 2 diabetes have found that they can reduce their hunger level by avoiding high-GI foods and by making sure that they don't eat large portions of carbohydrate-containing foods at any one meal or snack. Reducing the amount of carbohydrate that is on your plate while also adding some more low-carbohydrate vegetables and protein can help reduce your blood sugar response and keep you feeling full for longer.

A dietitian can help you work out the amounts of different foods you should be consuming. Measuring your blood glucose responses to different meals will also help you work out the amounts of different foods that you can eat that enable you to keep your blood sugar level under control.

dietary guidelines
eat regular meals based on low-GI foods

Eating four to six small meals and snacks based on low-GI foods, spread out evenly over the day, rather than two to three large meals, can help improve blood sugar control. Ask your dietitian for advice about scheduling your food intake with your medication and activity patterns. Learn which foods contain carbohydrate and how much they contain, so you can spread out your carbohydrate intake over the day. Try to avoid eating large amounts of carbohydrate at any one meal.

limit your fat intake

It is particularly important for people with diabetes to control their fat intake because a high-fat diet increases insulin resistance and the risk of weight gain and heart disease. People with diabetes have a very high risk of developing heart disease and therefore need to limit their intake of saturated fat, which is particularly high in foods such as fatty meats, pastries, takeaway foods, egg yolks and full-fat dairy products.

tips for lowering the GI of your diet

◆ Substitute high-GI foods that you eat regularly with lower-GI versions.

◆ Base your meals and snacks on nutritious low-GI foods.

◆ Dilute higher-GI foods, such as regular white rice, with lower-GI foods, such as lentils, barley or kidney beans.

◆ Don't overcook pasta, rice, noodles or potatoes until they are soft and soggy.

◆ Use stone-ground flour in baking recipes.

◆ Use low-GI dried fruits (such as apples, apricots, peaches, pears and prunes) in breakfast cereals and baking recipes instead of higher-GI varieties (such as raisins, sultanas and dates).

◆ Substitute regular soft drinks, cordials and flavoured yoghurt with diet or no-added sugar varieties.

Use low-fat cooking methods and choose low-fat dairy products, lean cuts of meat and poultry, and low-fat spreads. Include small amounts of healthier fats in your diet, such as monounsaturated fat (found in foods such as avocados, olives and olive oil) and omega-3 polyunsaturated fat, which don't increase your blood cholesterol level or worsen insulin resistance: use olive oil or canola oil as the main oil you cook with, and eat oily fish such as tuna, salmon, sardines and trout three to four times a week.

eat a variety of fresh fruit and vegetables, and legumes

Aim to eat at least two serves of fruit and five serves of vegetables each day, preferably low-GI varieties with different colours. These foods help you feel full and provide antioxidants that help protect your body from the toxic effects of excess blood glucose. If you are trying to lose weight, increase the proportion of low-carbohydrate vegetables in your meals, such as mushrooms, broccoli, cauliflower, spinach and zucchini (courgette), rather than having large amounts of starchy foods, such as potatoes, rice and noodles. Having a bowl of clear soup as a starter can also help prevent you from overeating your main meal.

Legumes, such as lentils, chickpeas and soybeans, are highly nutritious foods and are particularly good for people with diabetes. They are low-GI foods and provide antioxidants and soluble fibre.

limit your intake of sugar and sugary foods

Sugar doesn't cause diabetes and people with well-controlled diabetes don't have to avoid sugar completely, but they should treat it with caution. Adding a little sugar (or better still, fresh low-GI fruit) to a bowl of porridge or breakfast cereal won't raise your blood sugar very much, but soft drink or sweets in between meals will send it soaring.

Reduced-sugar products, such as cordials and jams, are readily available. These have a lower blood sugar effect than regular varieties, but should still be enjoyed in moderation. Some low-calorie sugar substitutes can be used to replace sugar in baking recipes and to lower the calorie content and glycemic effect of the dish. However, they are only beneficial if you eat sensible amounts of the reduced-sugar food.

limit your intake of salt

A high salt intake can raise your blood pressure, which increases the risk of heart disease and kidney disease. Avoid adding salt to your meals and look for reduced-salt or no-added salt versions of canned and packaged foods. Use herbs, spices, lemon juice and vinegar to add flavour to meals and snacks. Salad dressing made with a little olive oil and lots of vinegar can be added to rice or pasta salads to help lower the GI of the salad.

only drink alcohol in moderation, if at all

Alcohol contains a lot of calories and should be avoided if you are trying to lose weight or have poorly controlled diabetes. Moderate alcohol consumption is no more than one to two standard drinks in a day with some alcohol-free days each week. Choose low-alcohol beer or dilute wine and spirits with soda water or a diet soft drink. If you take insulin or tablets for your diabetes, then you must eat some carbohydrate (such as bread or low-fat crackers) whenever you drink alcohol to prevent hypoglycemia (a dangerous drop in your blood glucose level). Ask your doctor whether it is safe for you to drink alcohol if you are taking any medication.

resources

Each person with diabetes needs to work together with various health professionals to learn how to best manage his or her condition with diet, exercise and medications. Different genetic and metabolic factors mean that there is no one ideal diet or medical regimen that will suit all people with diabetes. Although you have to take responsibility for managing your condition, there is plenty of help available for people with diabetes and those at risk of the condition. If you are not happy with a particular health professional, then look around until you find one that you feel comfortable with. There are support groups and associations for people with diabetes, which can provide you with medical devices, books and referrals to specialist health professionals. Diabetes research is constantly providing new information, so consult your doctor and other health professionals regularly.

Dr Susanna Holt, PhD, Dietitian

low-GI staples

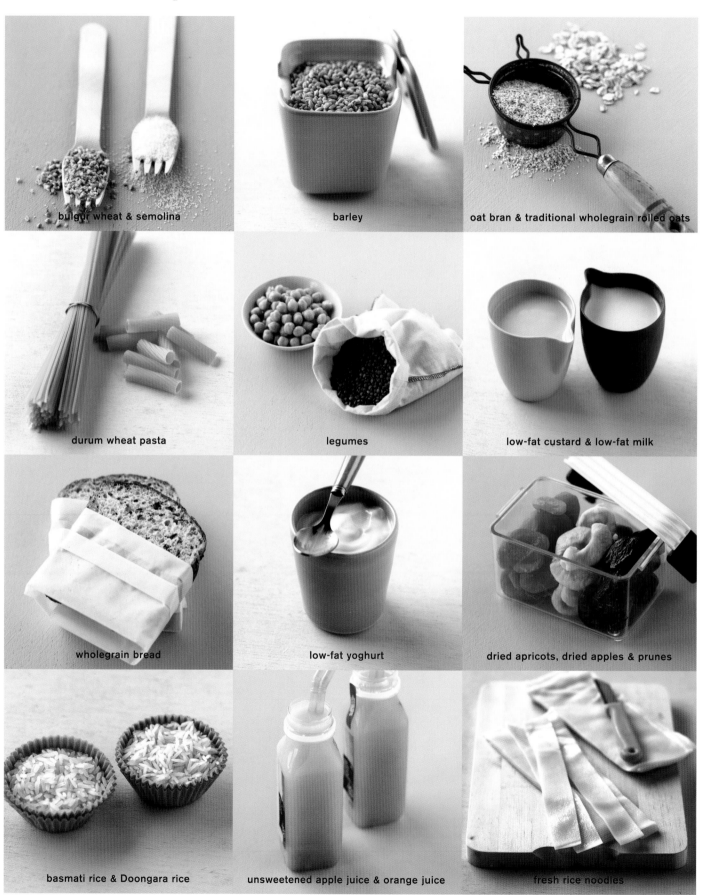

bulgur wheat & semolina

barley

oat bran & traditional wholegrain rolled oats

durum wheat pasta

legumes

low-fat custard & low-fat milk

wholegrain bread

low-fat yoghurt

dried apricots, dried apples & prunes

basmati rice & Doongara rice

unsweetened apple juice & orange juice

fresh rice noodles

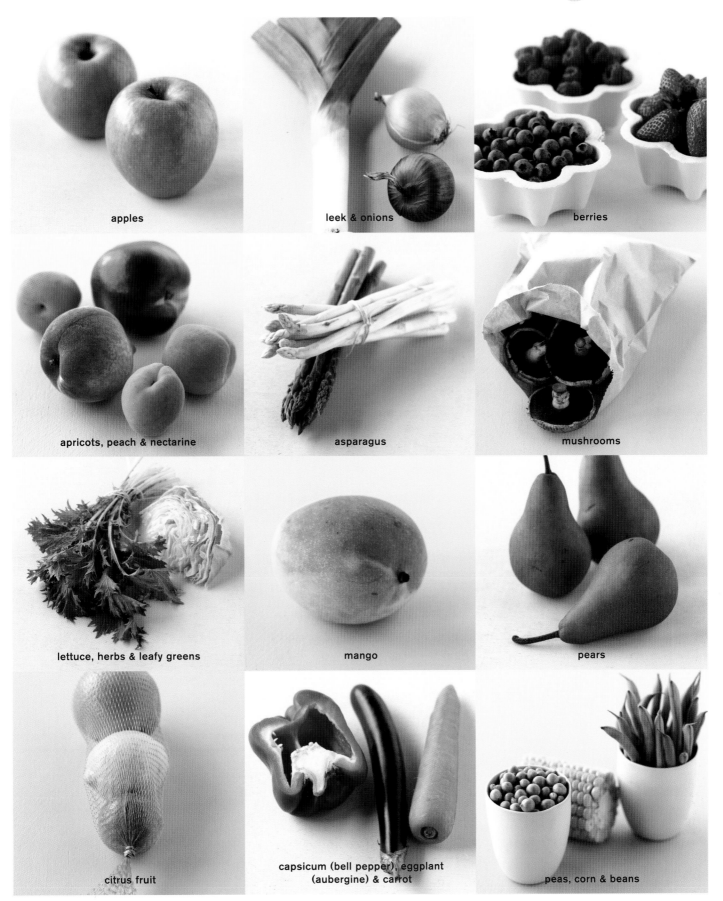

apples

leek & onions

berries

apricots, peach & nectarine

asparagus

mushrooms

lettuce, herbs & leafy greens

mango

pears

citrus fruit

capsicum (bell pepper), eggplant
(aubergine) & carrot

peas, corn & beans

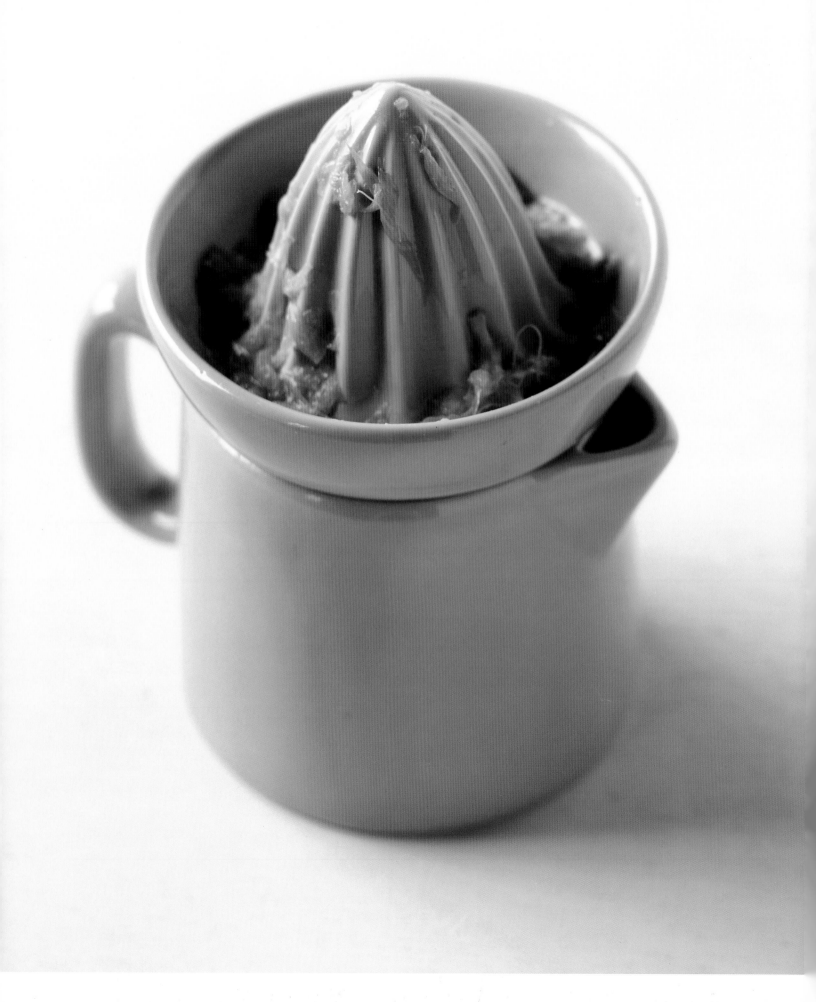

breakfast

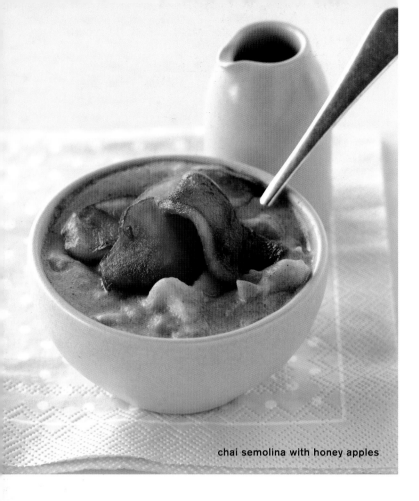

chai semolina with honey apples

ricotta pancakes with berries serves 4

250 g (8 oz) low-fat
  ricotta cheese
³⁄4 cup (185 ml/6 fl oz)
  low-fat milk
2 tablespoons
  unsweetened apple
  puree
1 cup (160 g/5¹⁄3 oz)
  stone-ground
  wholemeal plain flour

1 teaspoon baking
  powder
4 egg whites
olive oil spray
300 g (10 oz) fresh or
  frozen raspberries
1–2 tablespoons yellow
  box honey (optional)

1 Put the ricotta, milk and apple puree into a large bowl and mix to combine. Add the flour and baking powder and mix until just combined.

2 Whisk the egg whites in a clean, dry bowl until stiff peaks form. Slowly fold the egg whites through the batter. Do not overmix.

3 Lightly spray a non-stick fry pan with olive oil spray. Pour ¼ cup (60 ml/2 fl oz) of the batter into the pan and cook over medium heat for 3 minutes or until bubbles appear on the surface. Turn the pancake over and cook the other side until golden. Keep warm while you cook the remaining batter.

4 Serve the pancakes sprinkled with the raspberries and drizzled with the honey.

per serve fat 5 g ▌ saturated fat 1.5 g ▌ protein 17.1 g ▌ carbohydrate 44.8 g ▌ fibre 8.7 g ▌ cholesterol 2 mg ▌ sodium 290 mg ▌ energy 1307 kJ (312 Cal) ▌ GI low ▽

chai semolina with honey apples serves 4

1 teaspoon ground
  cinnamon
¹⁄2 teaspoon ground
  cloves
¹⁄2 teaspoon ground
  cardamom
¹⁄2 teaspoon ground
  nutmeg
¹⁄2 cup (80 g/2²⁄3 oz)
  semolina

100 g (3¹⁄3 oz) dried
  apples, finely chopped
2¹⁄2 cups (625 ml/
  20 fl oz) low-fat milk
2 apples, peeled and
  sliced
1¹⁄2 tablespoons yellow
  box honey

1 Put the ground spices, semolina, dried apples and milk into a pan. Stir over medium heat for 10 minutes or until the semolina is thick and smooth.

2 Put the sliced apples and honey into a pan. Cook over medium heat for 5 minutes or until the apples are soft and golden.

3 Spoon the semolina into 4 bowls and top with the honey apples.

per serve fat 0.8 g ▌ saturated fat 0.3 g ▌ protein 8.7 g ▌ carbohydrate 55.9 g ▌ fibre 4.9 g ▌ cholesterol 5 mg ▌ sodium 77 mg ▌ energy 1124 kJ (268 Cal) ▌ GI low ▽

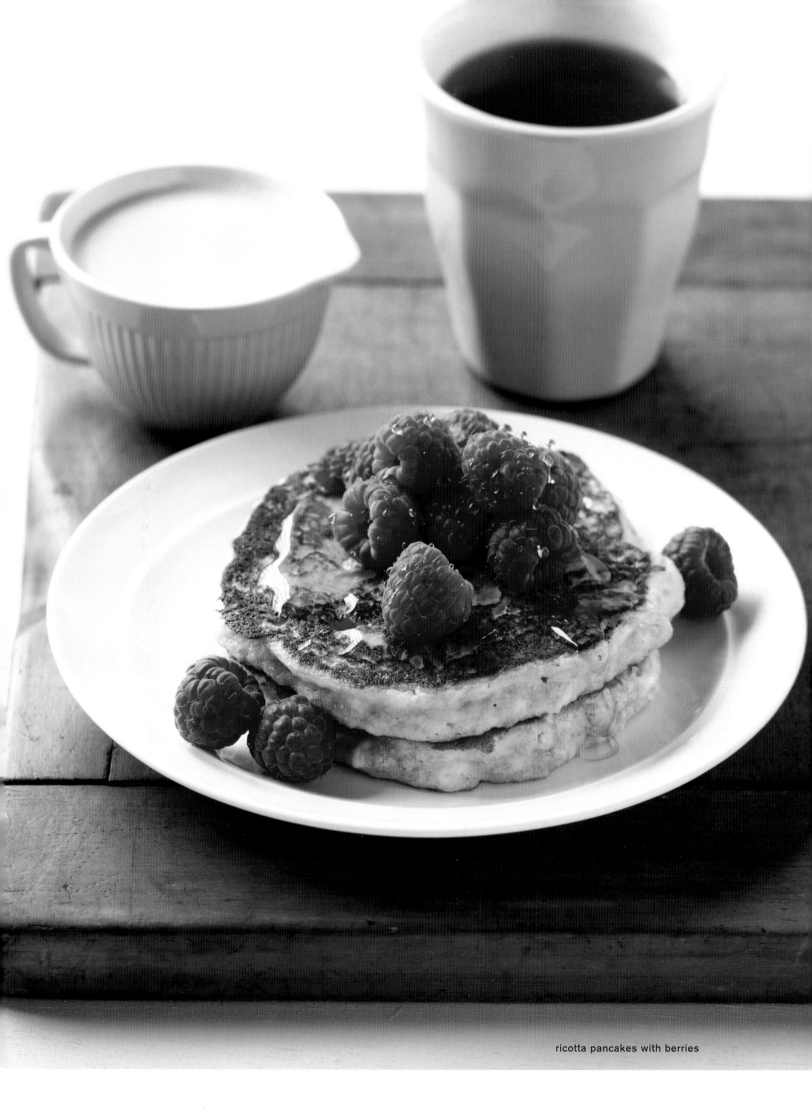

ricotta pancakes with berries

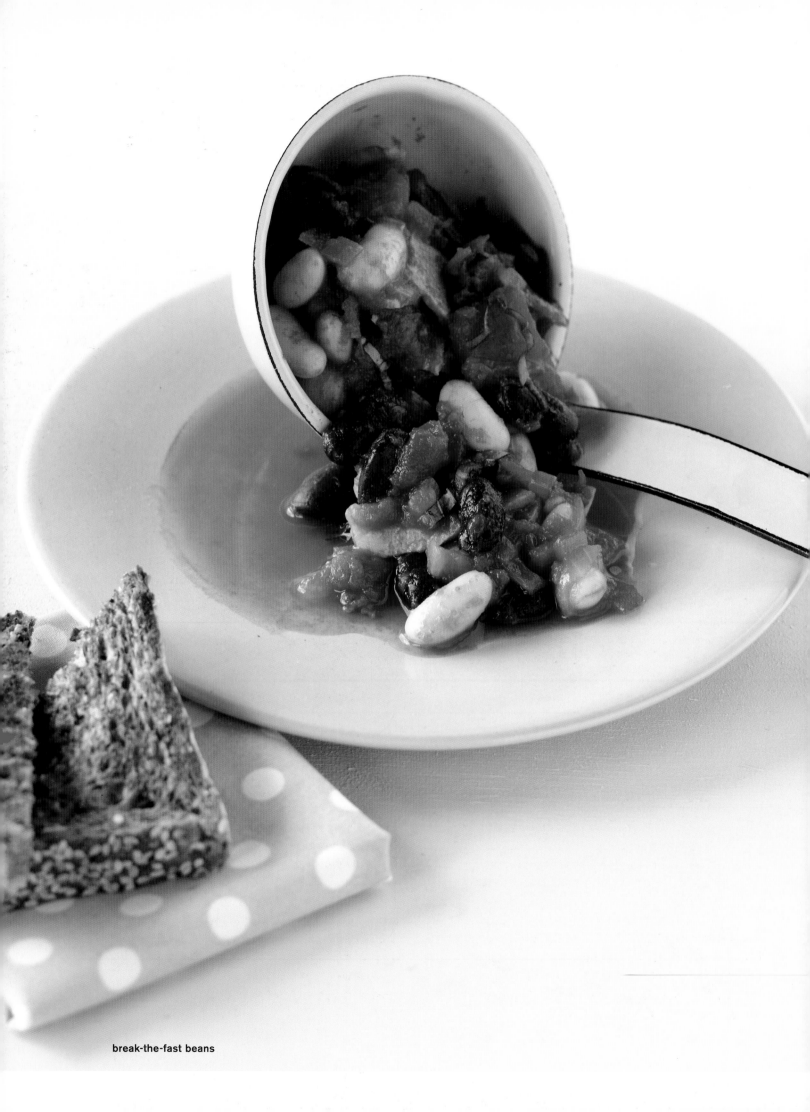

break-the-fast beans

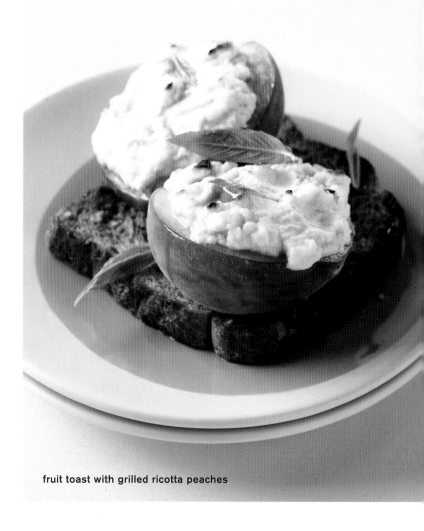

fruit toast with grilled ricotta peaches

break-the-fast beans serves 4

2 teaspoons olive oil
1 onion, chopped
100 g (3¹/₃ oz) 97% fat-free bacon, chopped
1 red capsicum (bell pepper), chopped
400 g (13 oz) can red kidney beans, rinsed and drained

400 g (13 oz) can cannellini beans, rinsed and drained
800 g (1 lb 10 oz) chopped tomatoes
2 teaspoons brown sugar
2 tablespoons finely shredded fresh basil
cracked black pepper

1 Heat the olive oil in a fry pan over medium heat. Add the onion and bacon and cook for 5 minutes or until soft and golden. Add the capsicum and cook for 3 minutes or until soft.

2 Stir in the beans, tomatoes and sugar. Bring to the boil and cook for 10 minutes or until the sauce has thickened.

3 Stir in the basil and season with cracked black pepper. Serve with toasted wholegrain bread.

per serve fat 4.1 g ▮ saturated fat 0.8 g ▮ protein 16.5 g ▮ carbohydrate 27.8 g ▮ fibre 11.2 g ▮ cholesterol 7 mg ▮ sodium 751 mg ▮ energy 966 kJ (231 Cal) ▮ GI low ▽

fruit toast with grilled ricotta peaches serves 4

4 freestone peaches
100 g (3¹/₃ oz) low-fat ricotta cheese
1 egg white, lightly beaten
1 teaspoon grated orange zest

1 teaspoon vanilla extract
4 thick slices dense wholegrain fruit bread
1 tablespoon pure maple syrup

1 Cut the peaches in half and remove the stones.

2 Combine the ricotta, egg white, orange zest and vanilla and spoon the filling over the peaches.

3 Place the peaches on a baking tray. Cook under a grill preheated to high for 3–5 minutes or until the peaches are soft and golden.

4 Toast the fruit bread until crisp and golden. Top with the peach halves and drizzle with the maple syrup. Garnish with mint leaves.

per serve fat 3.1 g ▮ saturated fat 0.8 g ▮ protein 8.2 g ▮ carbohydrate 37.5 g ▮ fibre 5.1 g ▮ cholesterol < 1 mg ▮ sodium 147 mg ▮ energy 939 kJ (224 Cal) ▮ GI low ▽

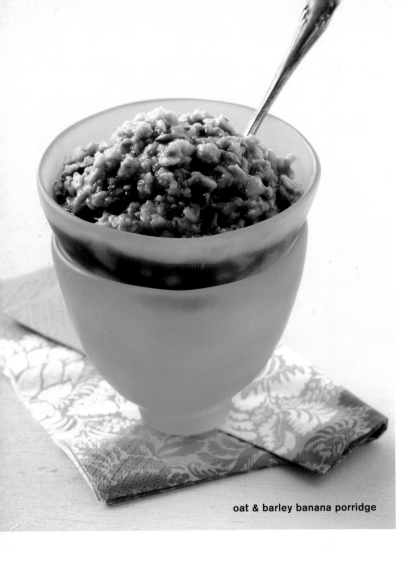

oat & barley banana porridge

oat & barley banana porridge serves 4

1 cup (100 g/3¹/3 oz)
  traditional wholegrain
  rolled oats
1 cup (100 g/3¹/3 oz)
  rolled barley
3 cups (750 ml/24 fl oz)
  water
2 tablespoons
  unprocessed oat bran

2 firm bananas, grated
1 tablespoon sunflower
  seeds
1 tablespoon pepitas
  (pumpkin seeds),
  roughly chopped
1 tablespoon pure maple
  syrup

1 Put the rolled oats, barley and water into a pan.
Cook over medium heat, stirring occasionally, for
5–10 minutes or until the porridge is soft and creamy.
2 Stir in the oat bran, bananas and seeds.
3 Divide the porridge among 4 bowls and drizzle
with the maple syrup. Serve with low-fat milk.
per serve fat 6.4 g ▯ saturated fat 0.9 g ▯ protein 8.2 g
▯ carbohydrate 52 g ▯ fibre 6.9 g ▯ cholesterol 0 mg
▯ sodium 3 mg ▯ energy 1248 kJ (298 Cal) ▯ GI low ▼

sardines on toast serves 4

4 slices wholegrain rye
  bread
200 g (6¹/2 oz) cherry
  tomatoes, squashed
  and drained
2 x 105 g (3¹/2 oz) cans
  sardines in spring
  water, drained

50 g (1²/3 oz) rocket
  (arugula)
1 tablespoon lemon
  juice
cracked black pepper

1 Put the bread slices on a baking tray and cook
one side under a grill preheated to medium until
golden brown.
2 Arrange the cherry tomatoes and sardines on
the untoasted side of the bread slices. Grill until the
sardines are browned.
3 Top the sardines with the rocket, sprinkle with the
lemon juice and season with cracked black pepper.
per serve fat 6.2 g ▯ saturated fat 1.5 g ▯ protein 14.5 g
▯ carbohydrate 22 g ▯ fibre 3.6 g ▯ cholesterol 51 mg
▯ sodium 309 mg ▯ energy 884 kJ (211 Cal) ▯ GI low ▼

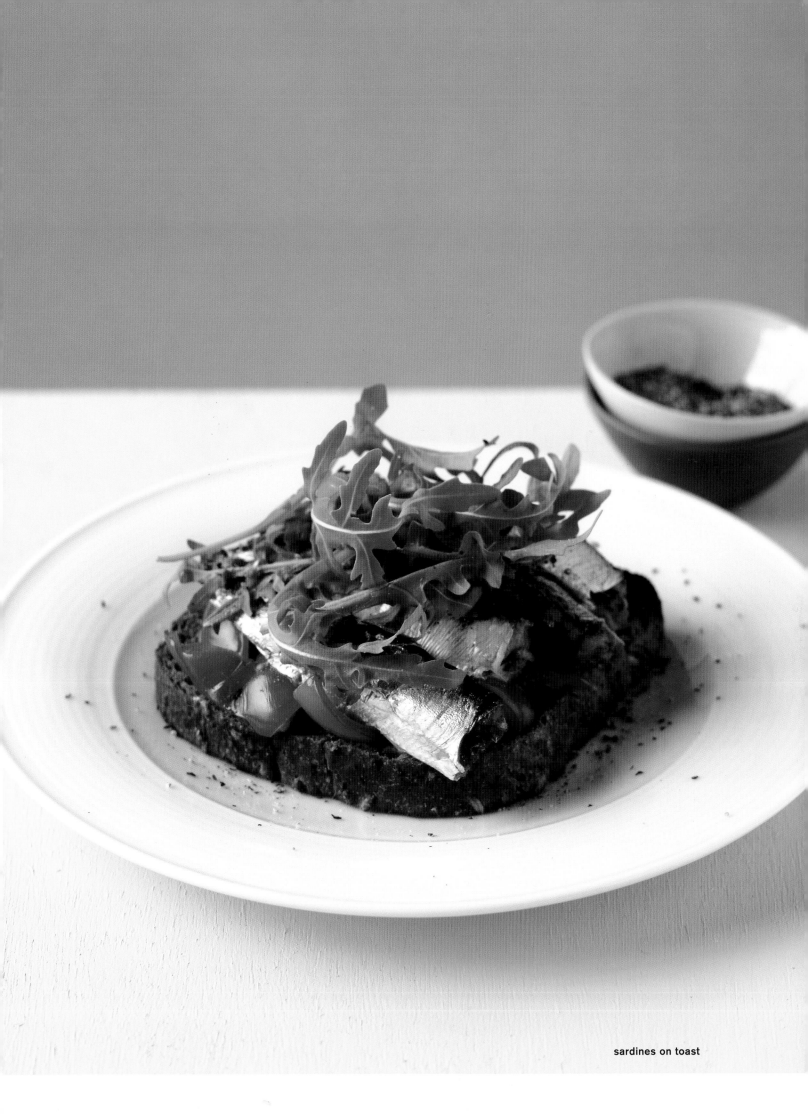

sardines on toast

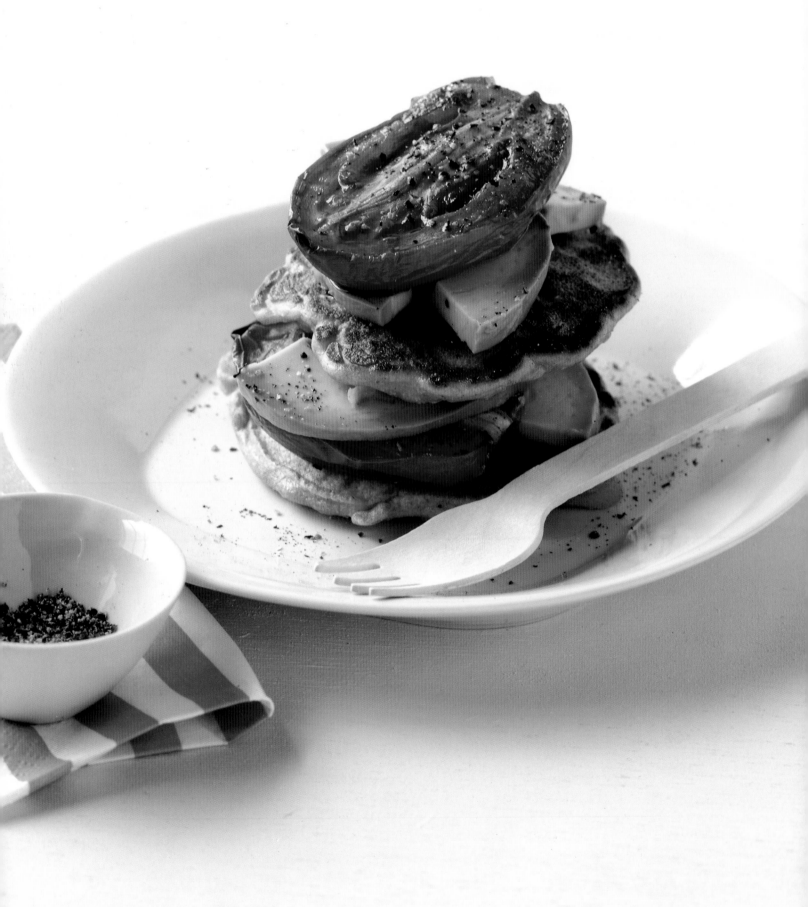

corn fritters with tomato & avocado

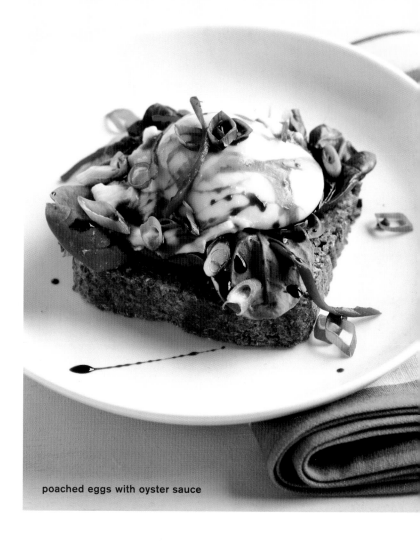

poached eggs with oyster sauce

corn fritters with tomato & avocado serves 4

4 Roma tomatoes,
  halved lengthwise
1 tablespoon balsamic
  vinegar
1 teaspoon brown
  sugar
cracked black pepper
1 cup (155 g/5 oz) fresh
  corn kernels
1 cup (170 g/5²/₃ oz)
  canned cannellini
  beans

2 tablespoons chopped
  fresh chives
2 teaspoons mild
  paprika
2 eggs, lightly beaten
½ cup (125 ml/4 fl oz)
  low-fat milk
½ cup (80 g/2²/₃ oz)
  stone-ground
  wholemeal self-raising
  flour
olive oil spray
1 small avocado, sliced

1 Preheat oven to 180°C (350°F/Gas 4).
2 Place the tomatoes on a baking tray, cut-side up. Drizzle with the balsamic vinegar, sprinkle with the brown sugar and cracked black pepper and roast for 30 minutes.
3 Put the corn kernels, cannellini beans, chives and paprika into a bowl and mix to combine. Stir in the eggs and milk, then fold the flour through the batter until smooth.
4 Lightly spray a non-stick fry pan with olive oil spray. Pour 2 tablespoons of the batter into the pan and cook over medium heat for 3 minutes on each side or until golden and cooked through. Keep warm while you cook the remaining batter.
5 Serve the fritters layered with the tomatoes and avocado and sprinkled with cracked black pepper.

per serve fat 12.9 g ▌ saturated fat 2.9 g ▌ protein 13.5 g
▌ carbohydrate 28.8 g ▌ fibre 8.8 g ▌ cholesterol 95 mg
▌ sodium 187 mg ▌ energy 1257 kJ (300 Cal) ▌ GI low ▼

poached eggs with oyster sauce serves 4

4 eggs
4 slices sprouted
  wholegrain (essene)
  bread
100 g (3¹/₃ oz) baby
  English spinach

2 teaspoons oyster
  sauce
1 large red chilli, thinly
  sliced
2 spring onions
  (scallions), sliced

1 Half fill a fry pan with water and place over medium heat until just simmering. Crack one egg at a time onto a plate and slide off the plate into the water. Reduce the heat to low and cook for 2–3 minutes or until done to your liking. Remove the eggs with a slotted spoon.
2 Meanwhile, toast the bread until golden. Top with the spinach and eggs. Drizzle the eggs with the oyster sauce and sprinkle with the chilli and spring onions.

per serve fat 7.1 g ▌ saturated fat 2.1 g ▌ protein 16.2 g
▌ carbohydrate 37.6 g ▌ fibre 9.1 g ▌ cholesterol 187 mg
▌ sodium 197 mg ▌ energy 1205 kJ (288 Cal) ▌ GI low ▼

breakfast

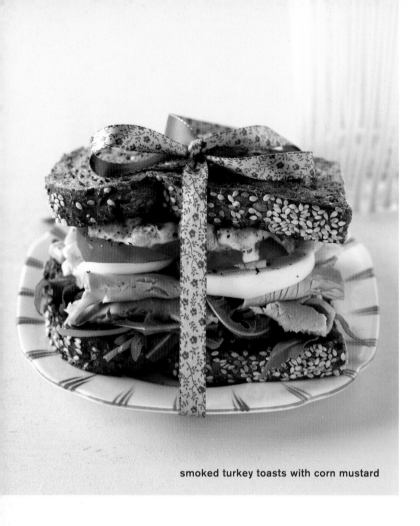

smoked turkey toasts with corn mustard

barley bircher with raspberry swirl serves 4–6

smoked turkey toasts with corn mustard serves 4

8 thick slices dense
    wholegrain bread
100 g (3^1/$_3$ oz) baby
    rocket (arugula)
200 g (6^1/$_2$ oz) smoked
    turkey slices
3 hard-boiled eggs,
    thickly sliced
2 tomatoes, sliced

200 g (6^1/$_2$ oz) can corn
    kernels, drained
2 tablespoons low-fat
    Greek-style plain
    yoghurt
2 tablespoons chopped
    fresh chives
1 tablespoon wholegrain
    mustard

1 Toast the bread until golden. Lay 4 slices of the toast on a flat surface. Top with the rocket, turkey, eggs and tomatoes.

2 Put the corn, yoghurt, chives and mustard into a bowl and mix to combine.

3 Spoon a large dollop of the corn mustard onto the tomatoes and finish with the remaining slices of toast.

per serve fat 9.1 g ▮ saturated fat 1.9 g ▮ protein 31.2 g ▮ carbohydrate 49 g ▮ fibre 7.2 g ▮ cholesterol 174 mg ▮ sodium 787 mg ▮ energy 1760 kJ (420 Cal) ▮ GI low ▼

2 cups (200 g/6^1/$_2$ oz)
    rolled barley
2 tablespoons
    unprocessed oat bran
1 teaspoon ground
    cinnamon
2 green pears, unpeeled,
    grated
1 cup (135 g/4^1/$_2$ oz)
    dried pears, chopped
^{1}/$_3$ cup (50 g/1^2/$_3$ oz) raw
    almonds, finely
    chopped

1 cup (260 g/8^1/$_3$ oz)
    low-fat Greek-style
    plain yoghurt
1 cup (250 ml/8 fl oz)
    low-fat soy milk
1 cup (250 ml/8 fl oz)
    unsweetened low-GI
    apple juice
1 teaspoon vanilla
    extract
250 g (8 oz) fresh or
    frozen raspberries

1 Put the rolled barley, oat bran, cinnamon, grated pears, dried pears, almonds, yoghurt, soy milk, apple juice and vanilla into a bowl and mix to combine. Cover and refrigerate overnight.

2 Put the raspberries into a blender and blend until fairly smooth.

3 Layer the muesli and raspberry puree in bowls.

per serve (6) fat 6.3 g ▮ saturated fat 0.6 g ▮ protein 10.2 g ▮ carbohydrate 59.6 g ▮ fibre 10.7 g ▮ cholesterol 2 mg ▮ sodium 57 mg ▮ energy 1422 kJ (340 Cal) ▮ GI low ▼

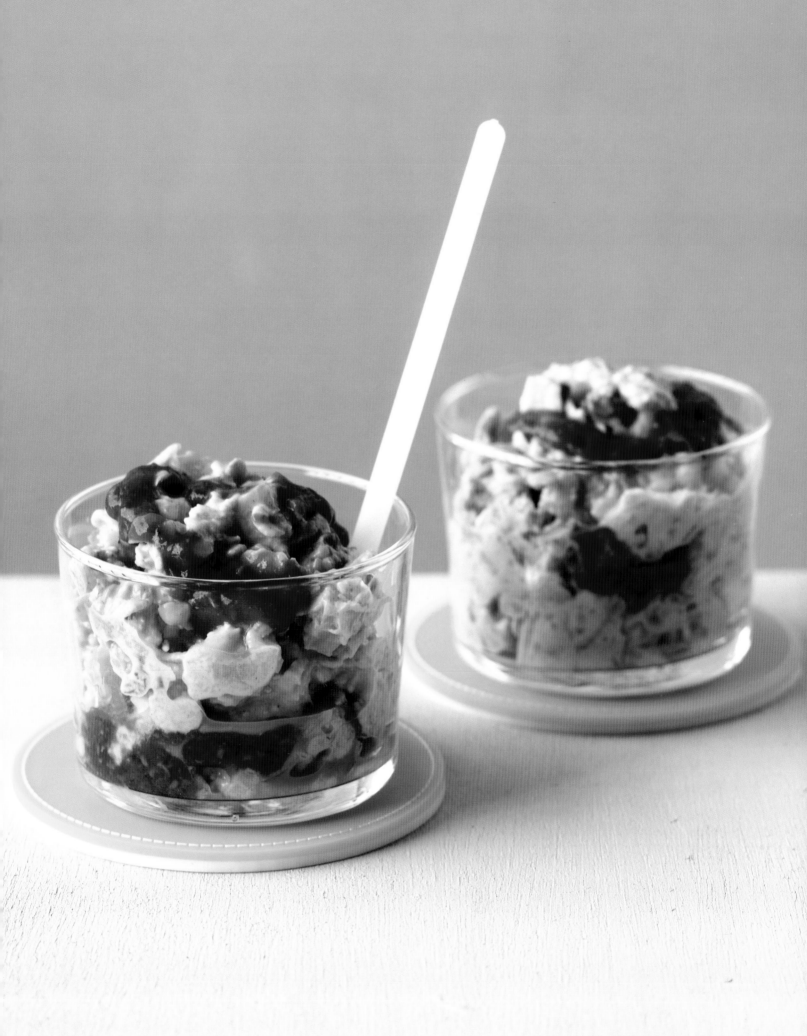

barley bircher with raspberry swirl

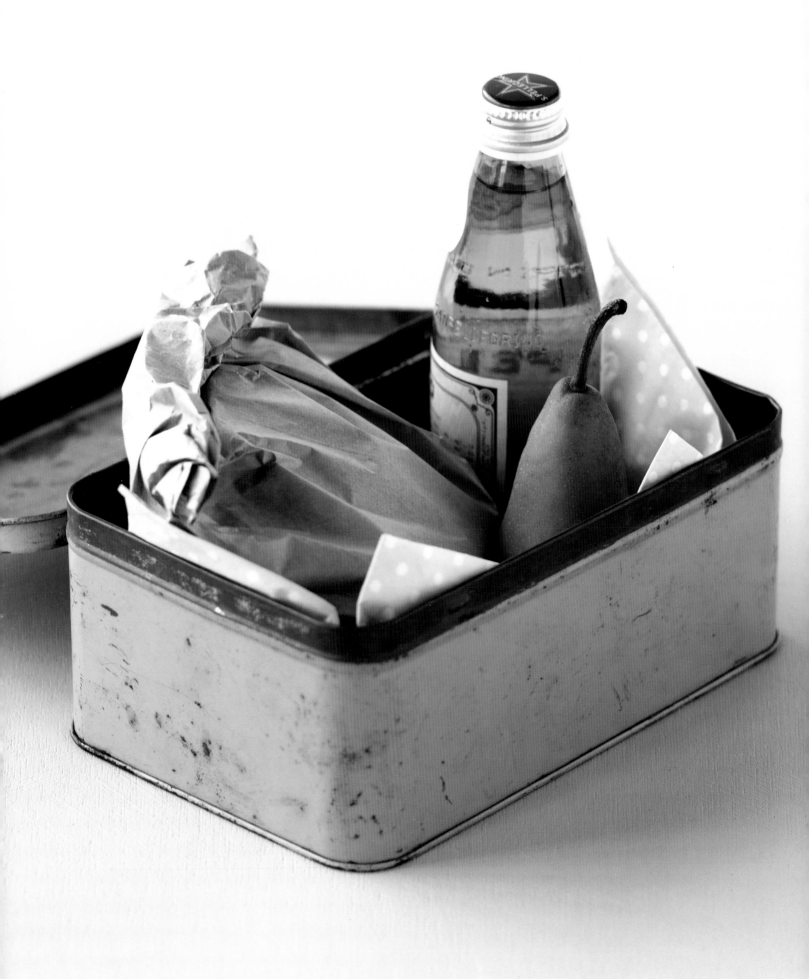

lunch

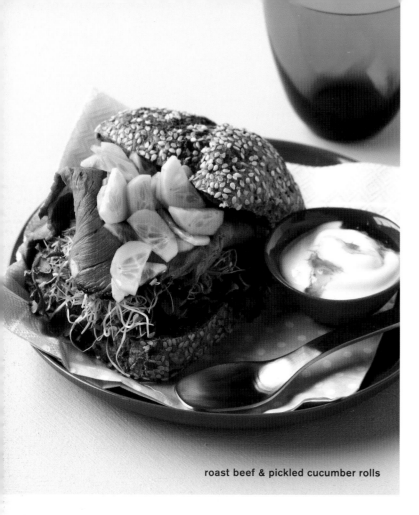
roast beef & pickled cucumber rolls

roast beef & pickled cucumber rolls   serves 4

2 Lebanese cucumbers, peeled

2 tablespoons rice wine vinegar

1 teaspoon sugar (optional)

100 g (3¹/₃ oz) watercress

30 g (1 oz) alfalfa sprouts

100 g (3¹/₃ oz) rare lean roast beef slices

4 wholegrain bread rolls, halved

2 tablespoons low-fat Greek-style plain yoghurt

2 teaspoons sweet chilli sauce

1 Cut the cucumbers in half lengthwise, then into thin slices. Put them into a bowl, add the vinegar and sugar and mix to combine.

2 Put the watercress, alfalfa and roast beef on the bases of the rolls. Add the cucumbers, a dollop of yoghurt and a drizzle of sweet chilli sauce. Replace the tops of the rolls.

per serve fat 3.4 g ▮ saturated fat 0.8 g ▮ protein 13.2 g ▮ carbohydrate 29.2 g ▮ fibre 4.7 g ▮ cholesterol 18 mg ▮ sodium 354 mg ▮ energy 892 kJ (213 Cal) ▮ GI low ▼

bean & vegetable soup with cheesy toasts   serves 4

2 teaspoons olive oil

1 onion, chopped

1 red capsicum (bell pepper), chopped

1 carrot, chopped

2 zucchini (courgette), chopped

400 g (13 oz) can chopped tomatoes

6 cups (1.5 litres/48 fl oz) reduced-salt chicken or vegetable stock

1 cup (200 g/6¹/₂ oz) broken durum wheat spaghetti

400 g (13 oz) can red kidney beans, rinsed and drained

250 g (8 oz) frozen spinach, thawed

100 g (3¹/₃ oz) green beans, sliced

2 thick slices wholegrain bread, cut into strips

¹/₂ cup (50 g/1²/₃ oz) grated parmesan cheese

1 Heat the oil in a large pan, add the onion and cook over medium heat for 5 minutes or until golden. Add the capsicum, carrot and zucchini and cook for 5 minutes or until the vegetables are soft.

2 Add the tomatoes and stock and bring to the boil. Add the broken spaghetti and cook for 5 minutes or until the spaghetti is soft.

3 Reduce the heat, stir in the kidney beans, thawed spinach and green beans and cook for 5 minutes or until heated through.

4 Put the bread strips on a baking tray and toast one side under a grill preheated to medium. Turn the bread over, sprinkle with the parmesan and grill until crisp and golden brown.

5 Serve the soup with the toasts to the side.

per serve fat 9.3 g ▮ saturated fat 3.4 g ▮ protein 22.9 g ▮ carbohydrate 64.8 g ▮ fibre 14.3 g ▮ cholesterol 34 mg ▮ sodium 1887 mg ▮ energy 1931 kJ (461 Cal) ▮ GI low ▼

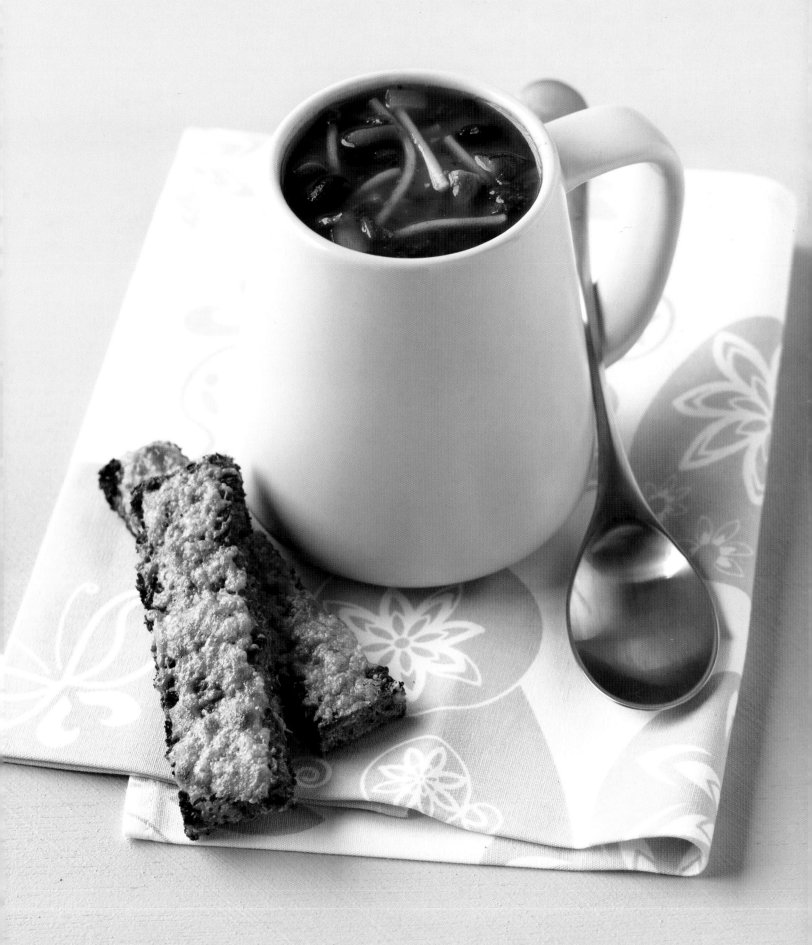

bean & vegetable soup with cheesy toasts

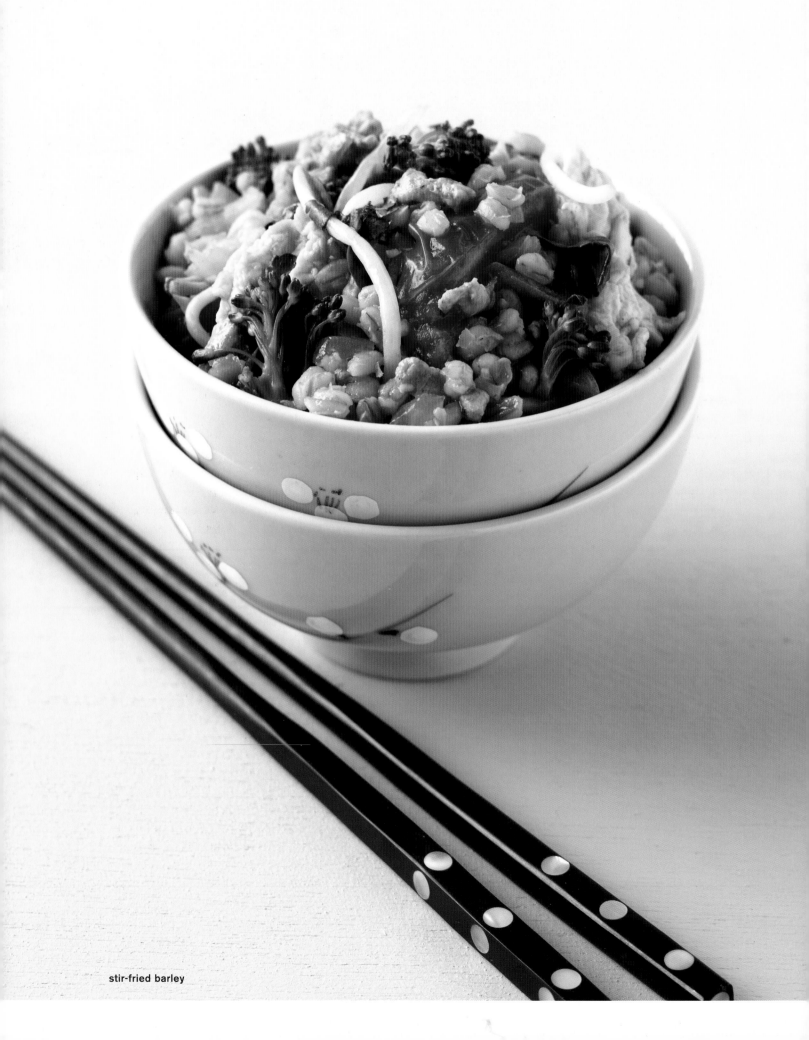

stir-fried barley

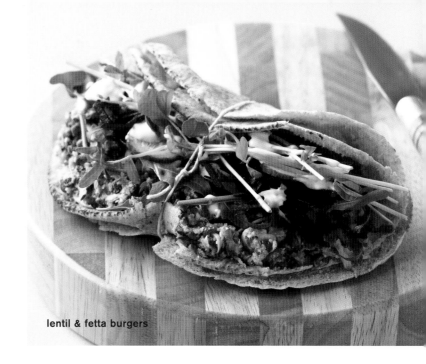

lentil & fetta burgers

stir-fried barley serves 4

1 cup (195 g/6¹/₂ oz)
  pearl barley

olive oil spray

2 eggs, lightly beaten

2 tablespoons water

1 teaspoon sesame oil

1 teaspoon olive oil

1 red (Spanish) onion,
  sliced

100 g (3¹/₃ oz) lean
  pork mince

2 cloves garlic,
  crushed

1 tomato, cut into
  wedges

200 g (6¹/₂ oz) broccolini,
  chopped

3 tablespoons chopped
  fresh coriander
  (cilantro)

100 g (3¹/₃ oz) bean
  sprouts

2 tablespoons fish sauce

1 tablespoon grated
  palm sugar or brown
  sugar (optional)

1 Cook the barley in a large pan of boiling water for 40 minutes or until just soft, adding more water if necessary. Rinse under cold water and drain well.
2 Lightly spray a wok with olive oil spray and heat over high heat. Whisk together the eggs and water, pour into the wok and cook until the eggs just start to set, then stir until scrambled. Remove from the wok.
3 Heat the sesame oil and olive oil in the wok, add the onion and stir fry for 3 minutes or until soft and golden. Add the pork and garlic and cook for 5 minutes or until the pork is browned.
4 Add the tomato and broccolini and stir fry for 3 minutes or until the broccolini is tender.
5 Add the barley, eggs, coriander, bean sprouts and combined fish sauce and sugar. Stir fry for 2 minutes or until heated through.

per serve fat 7.5 g ▍ saturated fat 1.7 g ▍ protein 17.5 g
▍ carbohydrate 36.6 g ▍ fibre 9.7 g ▍ cholesterol 113 mg
▍ sodium 990 mg ▍ energy 1271 kJ (304 Cal) ▍ GI low ▽

lentil & fetta burgers serves 4

400 g (13 oz) can brown
  lentils, rinsed and
  drained

50 g (1²/₃ oz) low-fat
  fetta cheese, crumbled

1 zucchini (courgette),
  grated

1 tablespoon fresh dill,
  chopped

1 egg, lightly beaten

¹/₂ cup (70 g/2¹/₄ oz)
  unprocessed oat bran

olive oil spray

4 small wholemeal pita
  breads

100 g (3¹/₃ oz) rocket
  (arugula)

50 g (1²/₃ oz) snowpea
  sprouts

2 tablespoons low-fat
  mayonnaise

2 tablespoons low-fat
  Greek-style plain
  yoghurt

1 beetroot, peeled and
  grated

1 Lebanese cucumber,
  unpeeled, sliced

1 Combine the lentils, fetta, zucchini and dill in a bowl. Add the egg and oat bran and mix well. Shape the mixture into 4 flat patties.
2 Lightly spray a non-stick fry pan with olive oil spray and heat over medium heat. Cook the patties for 10 minutes or until heated through, then turn and cook the other side.
3 Lay the pita breads on a flat surface. Top with the rocket, lentil patties, snowpea sprouts, mayonnaise, yoghurt, beetroot and cucumber.

per serve fat 6.4 g ▍ saturated fat 2 g ▍ protein 17.2 g
▍ carbohydrate 46.1 g ▍ fibre 10 g ▍ cholesterol 50 mg
▍ sodium 631 mg ▍ energy 1391 kJ (332 Cal) ▍ GI low ▽

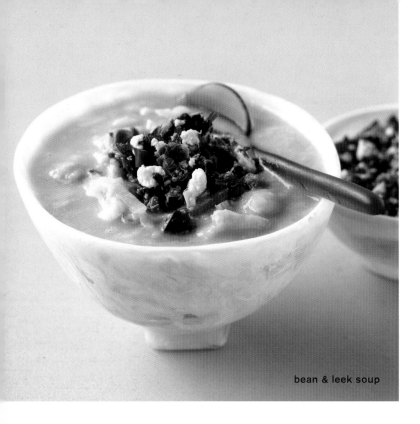

bean & leek soup

bean & leek soup serves 4

2 teaspoons olive oil

3 leeks, thinly sliced

400 g (13 oz) can
chickpeas, rinsed
and drained

400 g (13 oz) can
cannellini beans,
rinsed and drained

4 cups (1 litre/32 fl oz)
reduced-salt chicken
stock

2 tablespoons chopped
fresh flat-leaf parsley

2 tablespoons capers,
chopped

1 tablespoon chopped
kalamata olives

50 g (1²/₃ oz) low-fat
fetta cheese, crumbled

1 Heat the oil in a large pan over medium heat, add
the leeks and cook for 10 minutes or until softened.
Add the chickpeas and cannellini beans and cook for
3 minutes.

2 Add the stock, bring to the boil, then reduce the
heat and simmer for 25 minutes. Transfer half the
soup to a blender and blend until coarsely chopped,
then return to the pan and bring to the boil.

3 Put the parsley, capers, olives and fetta into a
bowl and mix to combine.

4 Spoon the soup into bowls and serve topped with
the parsley mixture.

per serve fat 6.1 g ▮ saturated fat 1.8 g ▮ protein 16.7 g
▮ carbohydrate 24.2 g ▮ fibre 9.2 g ▮ cholesterol 7 mg
▮ sodium 1017 mg ▮ energy 966 kJ (231 Cal) ▮ GI low ▼

salmon & rocket pasta salad serves 4

400 g (13 oz) thick
durum wheat tube
pasta

2 teaspoons olive oil

3 cloves garlic, crushed

400 g (13 oz) can
cannellini beans,
rinsed and drained

2 zucchini (courgette),
grated

1 iceberg lettuce,
roughly chopped

100 g (3¹/₃ oz) baby
rocket (arugula)

200 g (6¹/₂ oz) smoked
salmon, torn into
large pieces

2 tablespoons finely
shredded preserved
lemon

2 tablespoons lemon
juice

cracked black pepper

1 Cook the pasta in a large pan of rapidly boiling
water until al dente (cooked, but still with a bite to
it). Drain and transfer to a large bowl.

2 Heat the oil in a pan over medium heat. Add
the garlic, beans, zucchini and lettuce and cook for
5 minutes or until the lettuce has wilted.

3 Toss the lettuce mixture, the rocket and smoked
salmon through the pasta.

4 Gently fold the preserved lemon and lemon juice
through the salad and season with cracked black
pepper. Serve with lemon wedges.

per serve fat 6.5 g ▮ saturated fat 1 g ▮ protein 30.4 g
▮ carbohydrate 79.1 g ▮ fibre 11.5 g ▮ cholesterol 24 mg
▮ sodium 900 mg ▮ energy 2186 kJ (522 Cal) ▮ GI low ▼

▮ If you have high blood pressure, replace the
preserved lemon with grated lemon zest, which is
lower in sodium.

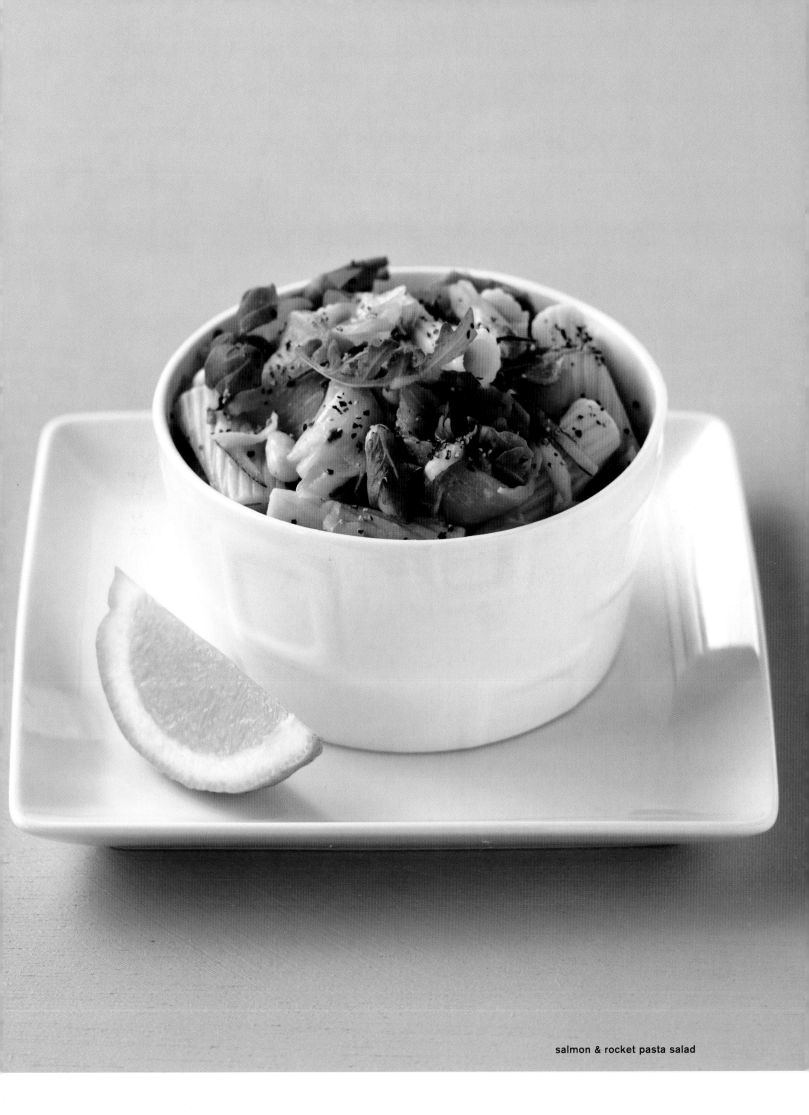

salmon & rocket pasta salad

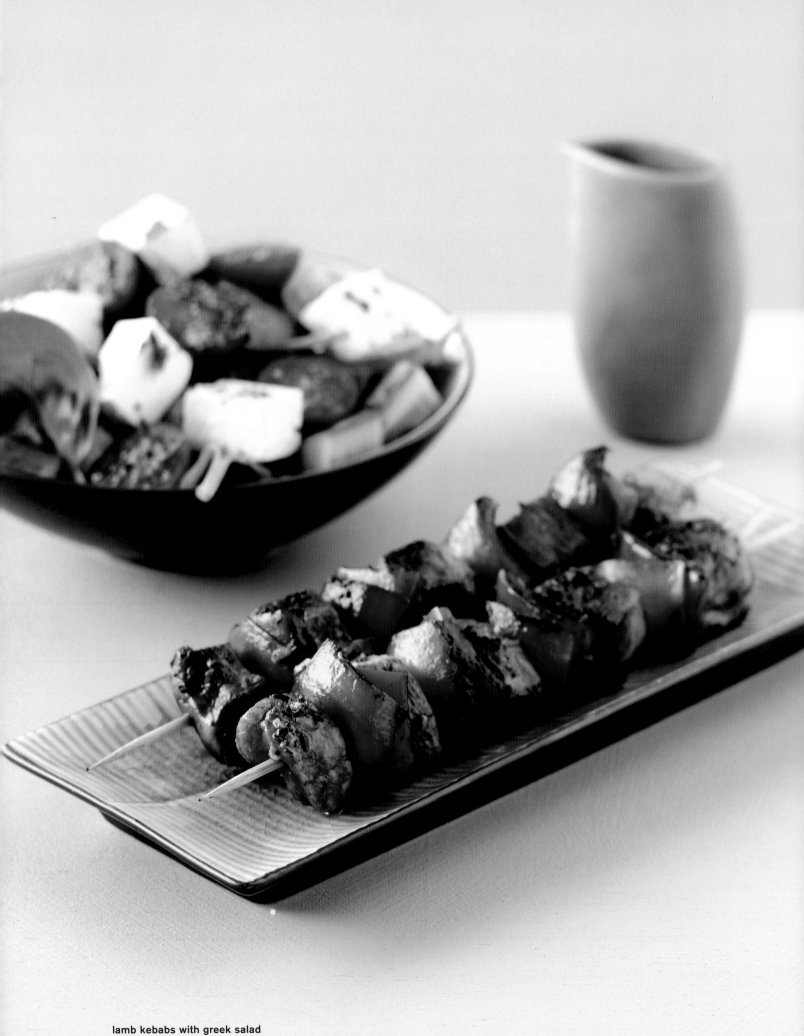

lamb kebabs with greek salad

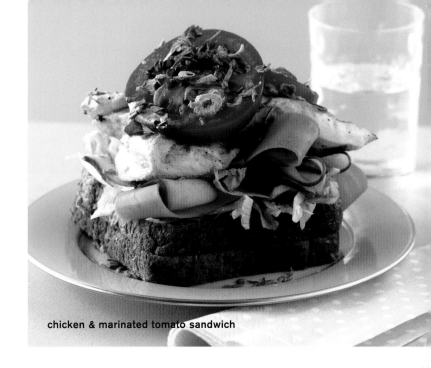
chicken & marinated tomato sandwich

lamb kebabs with greek salad serves 4

500 g (1 lb) lean lamb backstraps, cut into 2.5 cm (1 in) cubes

1 red capsicum (bell pepper), cut into squares

½ red (Spanish) onion, cut into squares

1 tablespoon balsamic vinegar

3 teaspoons olive oil

2 cloves garlic, crushed

1 teaspoon fresh rosemary, chopped

1 teaspoon fresh thyme, chopped

200 g (6½ oz) cherry tomatoes, halved

100 g (3⅓ oz) baby English spinach

1 Lebanese cucumber, unpeeled, chopped

50 g (1⅔ oz) low-fat fetta cheese, cubed

2 tablespoons lemon juice

1 teaspoon fresh lemon thyme, chopped

1 Soak 4 bamboo skewers in water for 30 minutes.
2 Thread the lamb, capsicum and onion onto the skewers and put in a shallow non-metallic dish.
3 Whisk together the vinegar, 1 teaspoon of the oil, the garlic, rosemary and thyme and pour over the lamb skewers. Cover and refrigerate for 30 minutes.
4 Put the tomatoes, spinach, cucumber and fetta into a bowl and gently toss to combine. Whisk together the lemon juice, remaining olive oil and lemon thyme and drizzle over the salad.
5 Preheat a lightly oiled barbecue flatplate or large fry pan. Cook the lamb kebabs for 5–10 minutes on each side or until done to your liking. Serve with the salad and a low-GI bread.

per serve fat 11.8 g ▌ saturated fat 4.6 g ▌ protein 29.7 g ▌ carbohydrate 3.9 g ▌ fibre 2.6 g ▌ cholesterol 85 mg ▌ sodium 268 mg ▌ energy 1039 kJ (248 Cal) ▌ GI low ▼

chicken & marinated tomato sandwich serves 4

3 tomatoes, thickly sliced

2 tablespoons red wine vinegar

1 teaspoon sugar

salt

2 tablespoons chopped fresh coriander (cilantro)

2 skinless chicken breast fillets

olive oil spray

8 thick slices wholegrain bread

1 cup (60 g/2 oz) shredded lettuce

50 g (1⅔ oz) snowpea sprouts

1 carrot, peeled into ribbons

1 Lebanese cucumber, peeled into ribbons

2 tablespoons fried onion flakes

1 Put the tomatoes into a non-metallic bowl. Drizzle with the vinegar and sprinkle with the sugar, salt and coriander. Set aside to marinate for 1 hour.
2 Slice the chicken breasts in half through the centre to give 4 thin pieces. Lightly spray a barbecue grill or large non-stick fry pan with olive oil spray. Preheat the grill or fry pan and cook the chicken for 5 minutes or until tender.
3 Lay 4 slices of the bread on a flat surface. Divide the lettuce, snowpea sprouts, carrot and cucumber among the bread. Top with the chicken and tomatoes. Drizzle with a little of the marinade, sprinkle with the onion flakes and finish with the remaining bread.

per serve fat 4.5 g ▌ saturated fat 0.8 g ▌ protein 33.3 g ▌ carbohydrate 39.6 g ▌ fibre 6.6 g ▌ cholesterol 70 mg ▌ sodium 427 mg ▌ energy 1465 kJ (350 Cal) ▌ GI low ▼

lunch

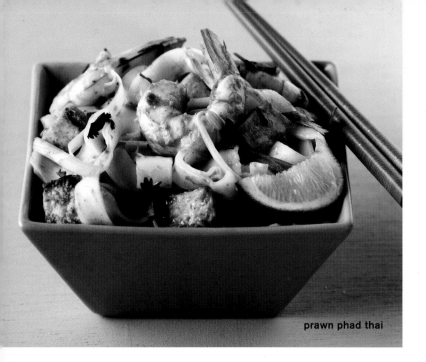

prawn phad thai

prawn phad thai serves 4

olive oil spray
200 g (6½ oz) firm tofu,
   cut into cubes
1 teaspoon chilli flakes
3 cloves garlic, chopped
2 teaspoons thinly sliced
   fresh ginger
300 g (10 oz) green
   prawns, peeled and
   deveined, tails left
   intact
2 tablespoons lime juice
1 tablespoon tamarind
   concentrate or puree
½ cup (125 ml/4 fl oz)
   water

1 teaspoon grated palm
   sugar or brown sugar
600 g (1 lb 3 oz) fresh
   rice noodles
4 spring onions
   (scallions), cut into
   short lengths and
   shredded lengthwise
3 tablespoons fresh
   mint, chopped
3 tablespoons fresh
   coriander (cilantro),
   chopped
100 g (3⅓ oz) bean
   sprouts

1 Lightly spray a wok with olive oil spray and heat over high heat. Add the tofu cubes and stir fry for 3 minutes or until golden. Add the chilli flakes, garlic, ginger and prawns and stir fry for 2–3 minutes or until the prawns are just cooked.

2 Reduce the heat and add the lime juice, tamarind concentrate or puree, water, sugar and noodles. Toss for 1 minute or until the noodles are soft.

3 Add the spring onions, mint, coriander and bean sprouts and stir fry for 1 minute. Remove from the heat and serve with lime wedges.

per serve fat 5.4 g ▮ saturated fat 0.6 g ▮ protein 21 g ▮ carbohydrate 67.5 g ▮ fibre 4.5 g ▮ cholesterol 56 mg ▮ sodium 187 mg ▮ energy 1743 kJ (416 Cal) ▮ GI low ▽

wild rice salad with mushrooms serves 4

125 g (4 oz) wild rice
½ cup (100 g/3⅓ oz)
   basmati rice
3 cups (750 ml/24 fl oz)
   water
6 dried shiitake
   mushrooms
2 tablespoons reduced-
   salt soy sauce
2 teaspoons sesame oil
¼ cup (60 ml/2 fl oz)
   mirin
1 tablespoon thinly
   sliced fresh ginger

100 g (3⅓ oz) mixed
   mushrooms (shiitake,
   Swiss brown, button),
   torn
1 tablespoon toasted
   sesame seeds
50 g (1⅔ oz) mung
   bean sprouts
2 spring onions
   (scallions), thinly
   sliced
30 g (1 oz) snowpea
   sprouts

1 Put the rice and water into a pan. Bring to the boil and cook for 20–30 minutes or until soft. The wild rice will still be slightly crunchy. Drain well.

2 Put the dried mushrooms into a bowl. Cover with boiling water and set aside for 10 minutes. Drain and thinly slice the mushrooms.

3 Put the soy sauce, sesame oil, mirin and ginger into a pan and bring to the boil. Add the soaked and fresh mushrooms and simmer for 3 minutes or until the mushrooms are heated through.

4 Stir the mushroom mixture into the rice. Add the sesame seeds, mung bean sprouts, spring onions and snowpea sprouts and mix to combine.

per serve fat 4.4 g ▮ saturated fat 0.6 g ▮ protein 9 g ▮ carbohydrate 44.1 g ▮ fibre 4.5 g ▮ cholesterol 0 mg ▮ sodium 378 mg ▮ energy 1120 kJ (268 Cal) ▮ GI low ▽

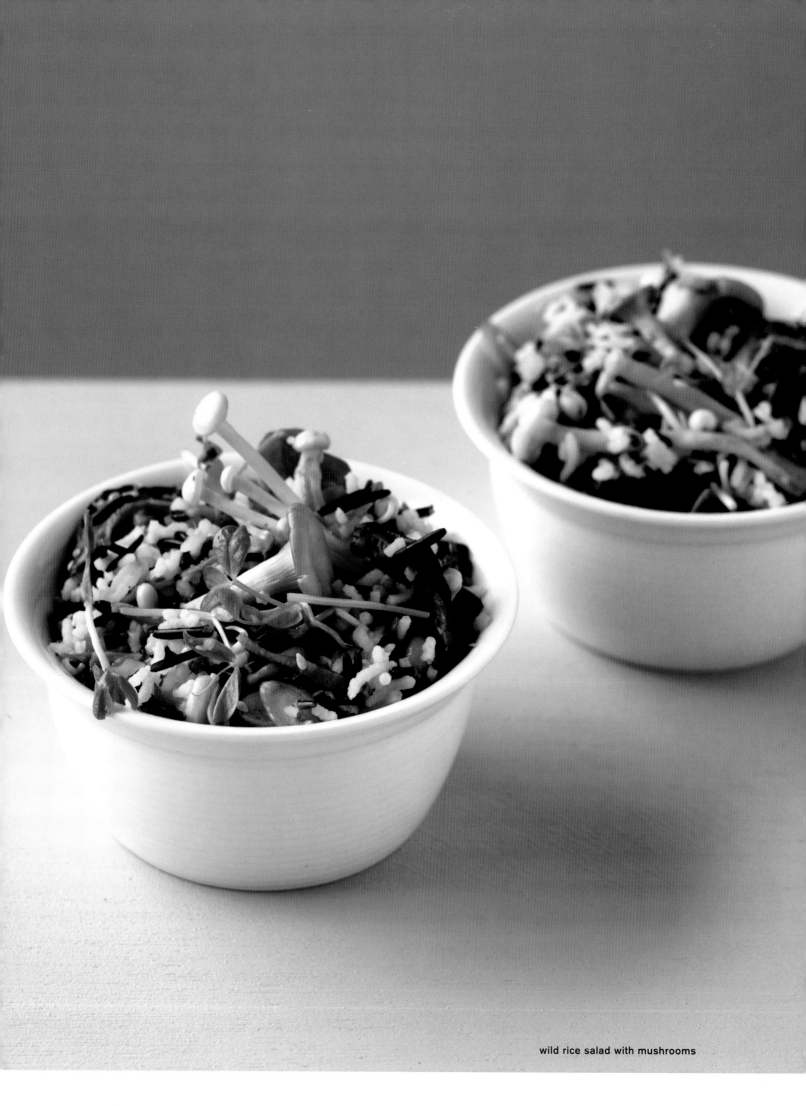

wild rice salad with mushrooms

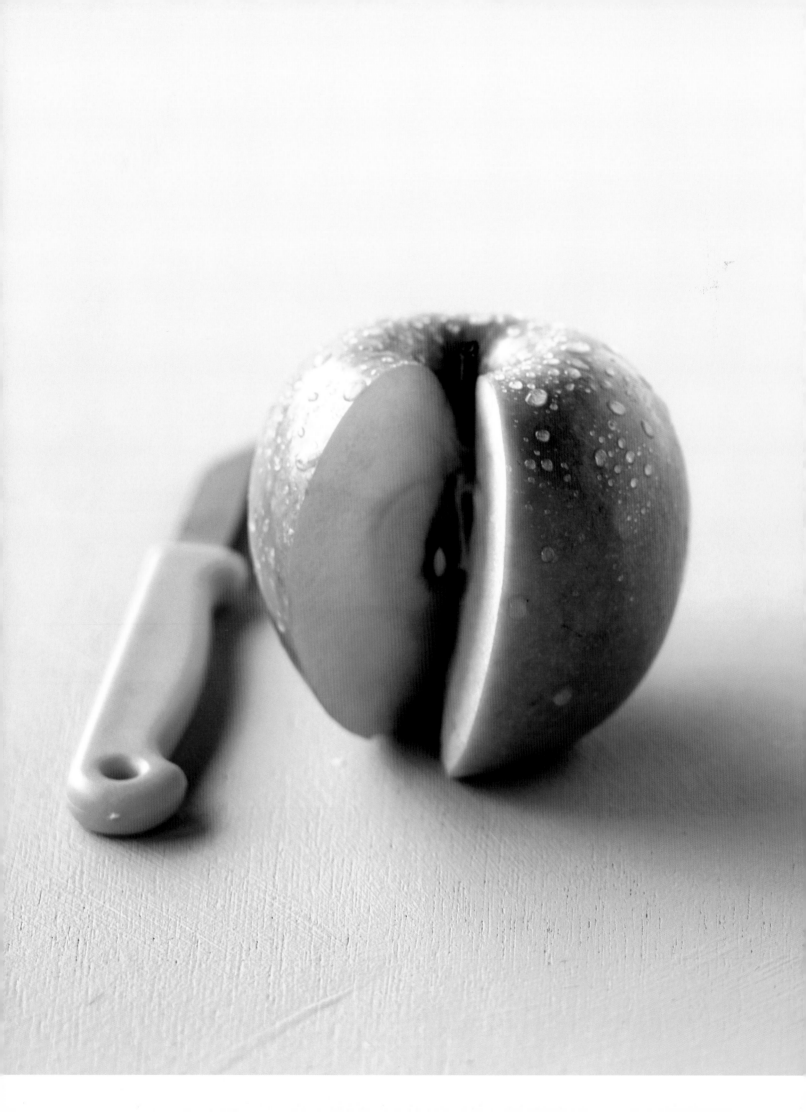

snacks

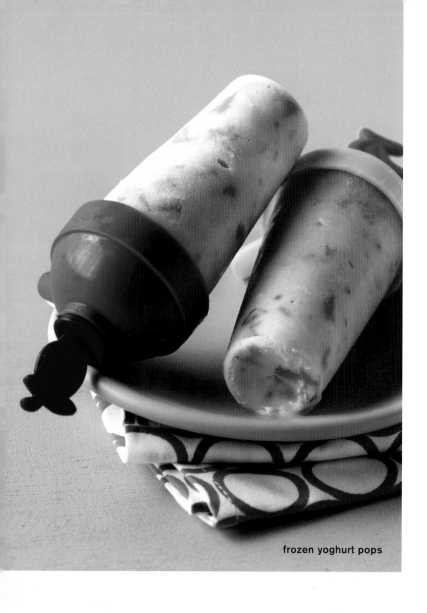
frozen yoghurt pops

frozen yoghurt pops makes 4

140 g (4¹/₂ oz) can diced
  peaches in mango
  juice
2 tablespoons toasted
  shredded coconut

2 cups (500 ml/16 fl oz)
  low-GI low-fat vanilla
  ice cream, softened
200 g (6¹/₂ oz) no-fat,
  no-added sugar
  apricot yoghurt

1 Put the peaches in mango juice, coconut, ice cream and yoghurt into a bowl and quickly mix to combine. Divide the mixture among 4 x ¹/₃ cup (80 ml/2²/₃ fl oz) capacity ice block moulds. Add the sticks and freeze until firm.

2 Rub a warm cloth around the base of each ice block mould and gently twist to release.

per yoghurt pop fat 4.2 g ▌ saturated fat 3.1 g ▌ protein 6.1 g ▌ carbohydrate 20.5 g ▌ fibre 0.9 g ▌ cholesterol 9 mg ▌ sodium 78 mg ▌ energy 608 kJ (145 Cal) ▌ GI low ▼

marinated artichoke & white bean dip serves 4

225 g (7 oz) drained
  marinated artichokes,
  rinsed to remove oil
400 g (13 oz) can
  cannellini beans,
  rinsed and drained

100 g (3¹/₃ oz) low-fat
  ricotta cheese
1 clove garlic,
  crushed
2 teaspoons tahini
1 tablespoon lemon
  juice

1 Roughly chop the artichokes and put into a food processor with the cannellini beans, ricotta, garlic, tahini and lemon juice. Process until smooth.

2 Spoon the dip into a bowl. Serve with toasted wholegrain bread and vegetables such as baby carrots, baby cos lettuce, celery and cucumber.

per serve fat 3.2 g ▌ saturated fat 0.7 g ▌ protein 9 g ▌ carbohydrate 10.4 g ▌ fibre 6.2 g ▌ cholesterol < 1 mg ▌ sodium 190 mg ▌ energy 487 kJ (116 Cal) ▌ GI low ▼

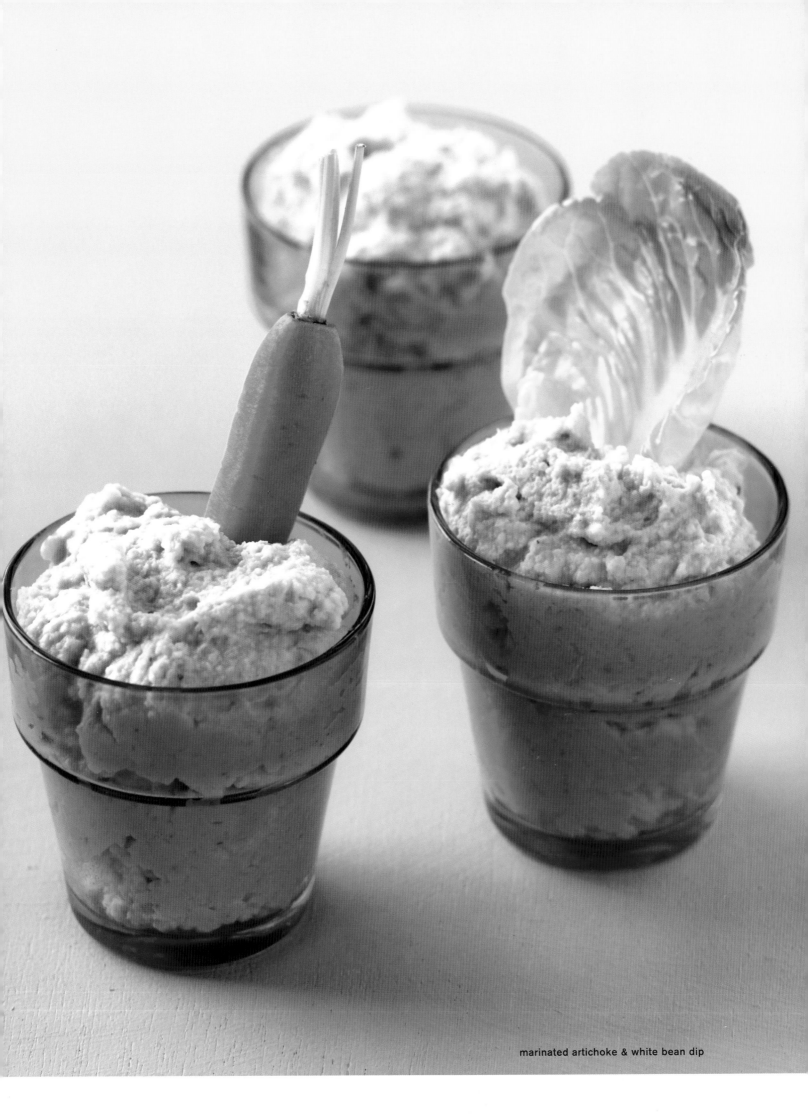

marinated artichoke & white bean dip

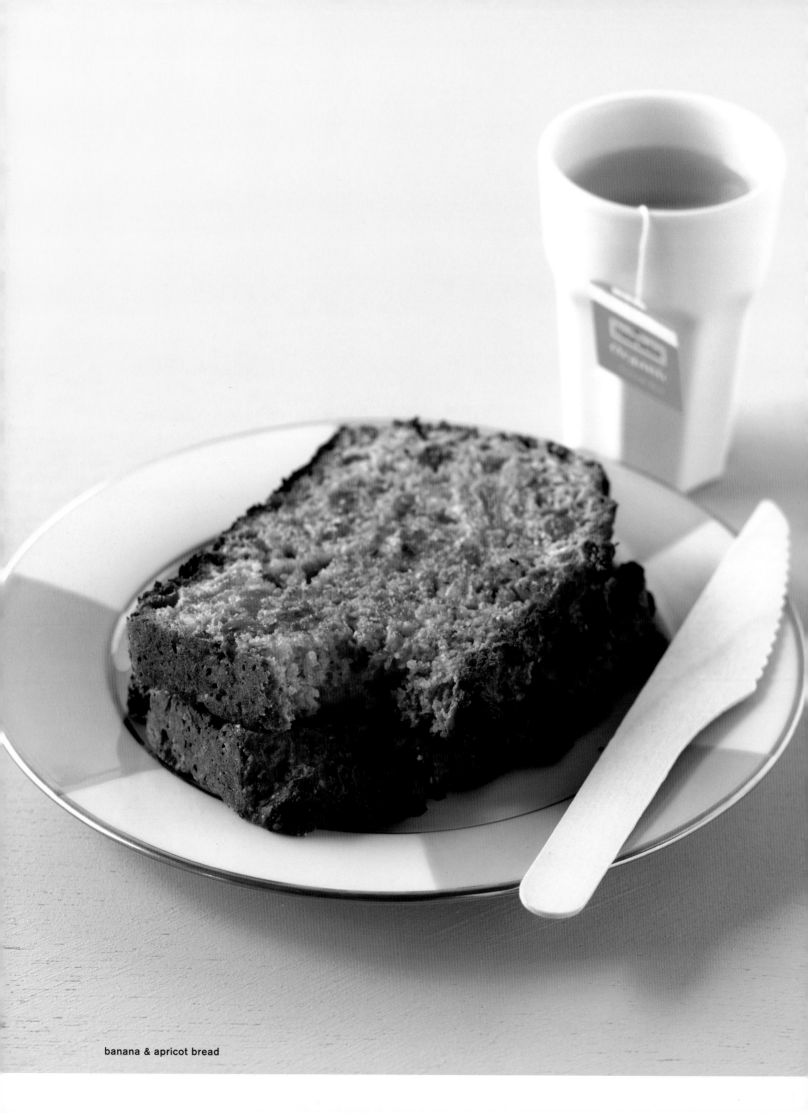

banana & apricot bread

banana & apricot bread serves 10

1 cup (135 g/4½ oz) dried apricots, roughly chopped

½ cup (85 g/2¾ oz) sultanas

1 cup (250 ml/8 fl oz) unsweetened low-GI apple juice

2¼ cups (360 g/12 oz) stone-ground self-raising flour

1 teaspoon baking powder

1 teaspoon mixed spice

½ cup (70 g/2¼ oz) unprocessed oat bran

3 tablespoons brown sugar or low-calorie sweetener suitable for baking

2 eggs, lightly beaten

1 cup (250 ml/8 fl oz) buttermilk

2 tablespoons olive oil

1 cup (240 g/7⅔ oz) mashed just-ripe banana

1 Preheat oven to 180°C (350°F/Gas 4). Lightly grease and line a 10 cm x 20 cm (4 in x 8 in) loaf tin.
2 Put the apricots, sultanas and apple juice into a pan. Bring to the boil and cook for 10 minutes or until the fruit has absorbed all the liquid.
3 Sift the flour, baking powder and mixed spice into a bowl. Stir in the oat bran and sugar or sweetener.
4 Whisk together the eggs, buttermilk and oil and stir into the dry ingredients. Fold in the mashed banana and fruit mixture.
5 Spoon the mixture into the prepared tin. Bake for 50–60 minutes or until a skewer comes out clean when inserted into the centre. Set aside for 5 minutes before turning out on a wire rack to cool completely. Serve the bread plain or toasted with a low-fat spread.

per serve (sugar) fat 6.2 g ▍ saturated fat 1.3 g ▍ protein 8.4 g ▍ carbohydrate 54.1 g ▍ fibre 4.6 g ▍ cholesterol 40 mg ▍ sodium 345 mg ▍ energy 1314 kJ (314 Cal) ▍ GI low ▼

per serve (sweetener) fat 6.2 g ▍ saturated fat 1.3 g ▍ protein 8.4 g ▍ carbohydrate 50.9 g ▍ fibre 4.6 g ▍ cholesterol 40 mg ▍ sodium 344 mg ▍ energy 1263 kJ (302 Cal) ▍ GI low ▼

▍ Enjoy in moderation as an occasional treat.

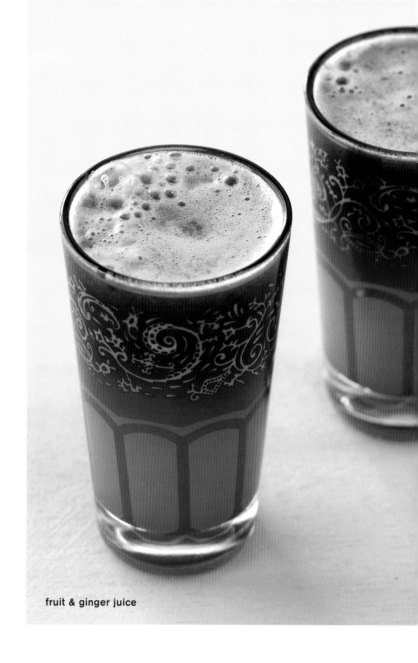
fruit & ginger juice

fruit & ginger juice serves 4

4 green apples, unpeeled

4 carrots, unpeeled

4 oranges, peeled and quartered

200 g (6½ oz) fresh or frozen blueberries

5 cm (2 in) piece fresh ginger

1 Push the apples, carrots, oranges, blueberries and ginger through a juice extractor.
2 Pour the juice into 4 tall chilled glasses and serve immediately.

per serve fat 0.4 g ▍ saturated fat 0 g ▍ protein 2.6 g ▍ carbohydrate 37.5 g ▍ fibre 8.5 g ▍ cholesterol 0 mg ▍ sodium 32 mg ▍ energy 752 kJ (180 Cal) ▍ GI low ▼

▍ Enjoy fruit juice in moderation, not as a daily drink.

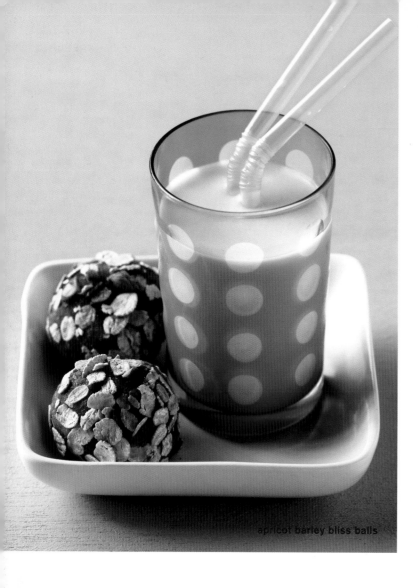
apricot barley bliss balls

spinach & ricotta pillows makes 12

100 g (3¹/₃ oz) baby English spinach	2 tablespoons grated parmesan cheese
75 g (2¹/₂ oz) low-fat ricotta cheese	cracked black pepper
	12 won ton wrappers
	olive oil spray

1 Preheat oven to 200°C (400°F/Gas 6). Line a baking tray with baking paper.

2 Wash the spinach and put into a pan. Cover and cook over medium heat for 5 minutes or until wilted. Cool slightly, then squeeze out any moisture and finely chop.

3 Put the chopped spinach, ricotta and parmesan into a bowl and mix to combine. Season with cracked black pepper.

4 Place 1 teaspoon of the filling in the centre of each won ton wrapper, brush the edges with water and fold over to form a triangle. Press the edges with a fork to seal.

5 Place the pillows on the prepared tray and lightly spray with olive oil spray. Bake for 15 minutes or until crisp and golden.

per pillow fat 1.1 g ▍ saturated fat 0.4 g ▍ protein 2 g ▍ carbohydrate 4.8 g ▍ fibre 0.4 g ▍ cholesterol 2 mg ▍ sodium 71 mg ▍ energy 163 kJ (39 Cal) ▍ GI low−med ▼−◆

apricot barley bliss balls makes 14

200 g (6¹/₂ oz) dried apricots, roughly chopped	1 tablespoon roughly chopped pepitas (pumpkin seeds)
200 g (6¹/₂ oz) dried pears, roughly chopped	¹/₂ teaspoon ground cinnamon
¹/₂ cup (50 g/1²/₃ oz) rolled barley	1 teaspoon brown sugar

1 Put the apricots and pears into a food processor and process to form a stiff paste.

2 Shape tablespoons of the mixture into balls and roll in the combined rolled barley, pepitas, cinnamon and sugar. Shake off any excess.

per ball fat 0.5 g ▍ saturated fat 0.1 g ▍ protein 1.3 g ▍ carbohydrate 18 g ▍ fibre 3.2 g ▍ cholesterol 0 mg ▍ sodium 7 mg ▍ energy 352 kJ (84 Cal) ▍ GI low ▼

▍ Enjoy in moderation as an occasional treat.

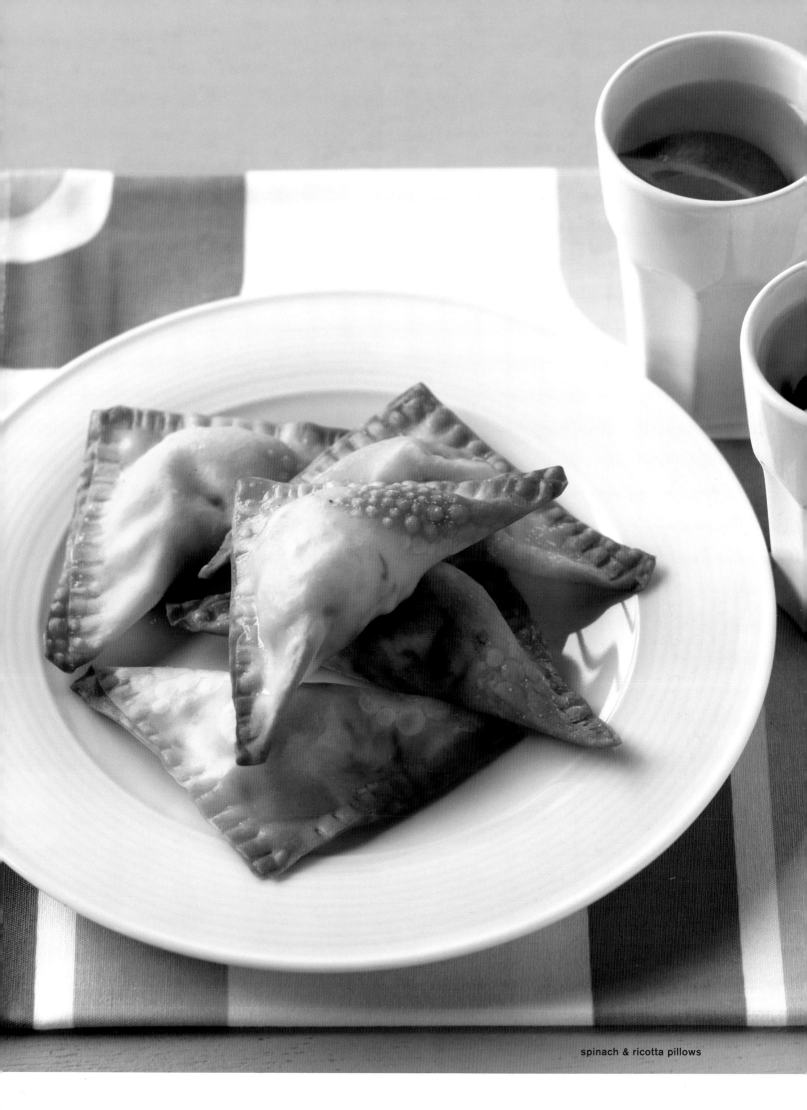

spinach & ricotta pillows

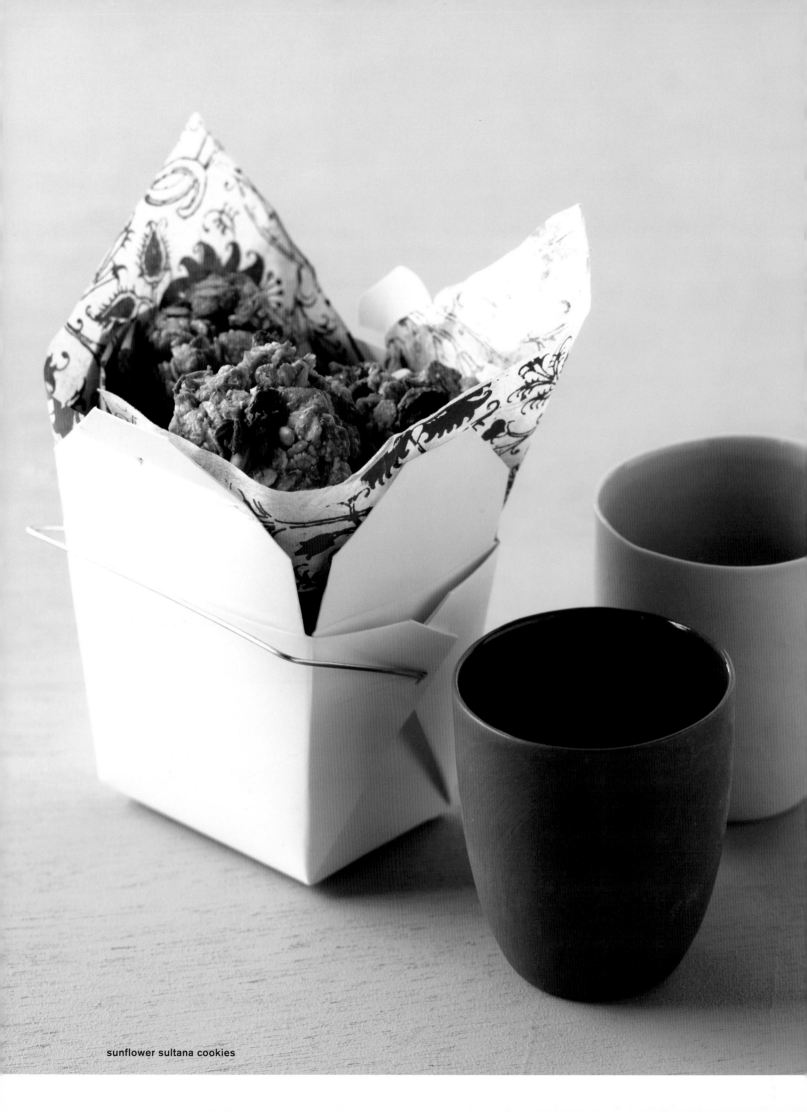

sunflower sultana cookies

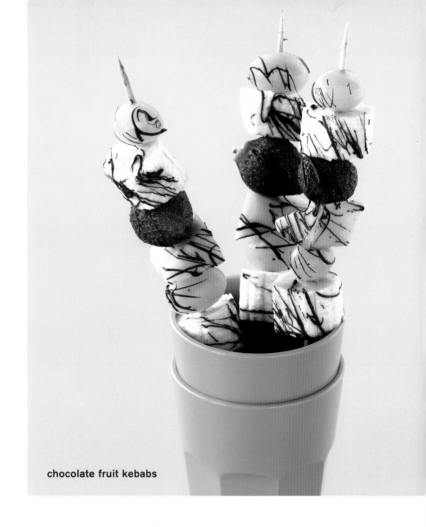

chocolate fruit kebabs

sunflower sultana cookies makes 12

1¹/₂ cups (150 g/5 oz) rolled barley

³/₄ cup (120 g/4 oz) stone-ground wholemeal plain flour

¹/₂ teaspoon ground ginger

¹/₄ cup (40 g/1¹/₃ oz) sunflower seeds

¹/₄ cup (45 g/1¹/₂ oz) sultanas

1 tablespoon crystallised ginger, chopped

1 tablespoon olive oil

2 tablespoons yellow box honey

³/₄ cup (185 ml/6 fl oz) unsweetened low-GI apple juice

1 Preheat oven to 180°C (350°F/Gas 4). Line a baking tray with baking paper.
2 Put the rolled barley, flour and ground ginger into a bowl and mix to combine. Stir in the sunflower seeds, sultanas and chopped ginger.
3 Whisk together the oil, honey and apple juice. Pour into the dry ingredients and mix well to combine.
4 Drop tablespoons of the mixture onto the prepared tray and flatten slightly. Bake for 15 minutes or until golden. Transfer to a wire rack to cool.

per cookie fat 3.7 g ‖ saturated fat 0.4 g ‖ protein 3.1 g ‖ carbohydrate 25.2 g ‖ fibre 2.9 g ‖ cholesterol 0 mg ‖ sodium 5 mg ‖ energy 604 kJ (144 Cal) ‖ GI low ▼

‖ You can replace the crystallised ginger with chopped dried pears to lower the sugar content and GI of the cookies.

chocolate fruit kebabs makes 4

100 g (3¹/₃ oz) seedless green grapes

1 just-ripe banana, thickly sliced

100 g (3¹/₃ oz) strawberries, hulled

1 firm ripe mango, cut into chunks

25 g (1 oz) dark chocolate, chopped

1 Thread the grapes, banana, strawberries and mango onto 4 bamboo skewers. Put the skewers on a baking tray lined with baking paper.
2 Put the chocolate in a heatproof bowl over simmering water. Do not let the base of the bowl touch the water. Stir over low heat until the chocolate has melted. Use a fork to drizzle the chocolate over the kebabs.
3 Place the tray into the freezer for 10 minutes or until the chocolate has set. Transfer to an airtight container and refrigerate until ready to eat.

per kebab fat 2.1 g ‖ saturated fat 1.7 g ‖ protein 1.8 g ‖ carbohydrate 19.5 g ‖ fibre 2.4 g ‖ cholesterol < 1 mg ‖ sodium 7 mg ‖ energy 448 kJ (107 Cal) ‖ GI low ▼

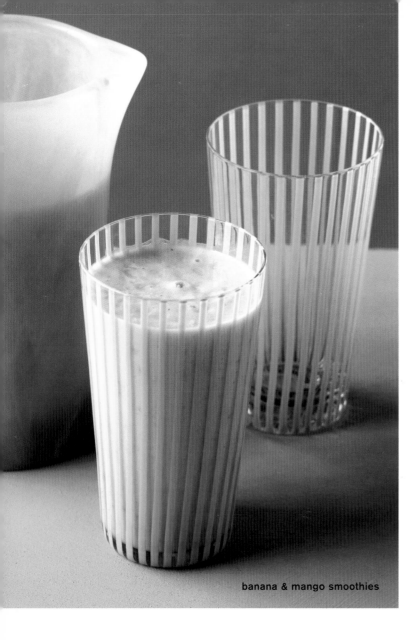

banana & mango smoothies

carrot & blueberry crumble muffins makes 10

1 cup (160 g/5^{1}/$_3$ oz)
   stone-ground
   wholemeal self-raising
   flour
^{1}/$_2$ cup (80 g/2^{2}/$_3$ oz)
   stone-ground self-
   raising flour
1 teaspoon ground
   cinnamon
^{1}/$_2$ cup (70 g/2^{1}/$_4$ oz)
   unprocessed oat bran
2 tablespoons brown
   sugar or low-calorie
   sweetener suitable
   for baking

1 carrot, grated
200 g (6^{1}/$_2$ oz)
   blueberries
1 egg, lightly beaten
^{1}/$_2$ cup (125 ml/4 fl oz)
   buttermilk
140 g (4^{1}/$_2$ oz)
   unsweetened apple
   puree
1 tablespoon olive oil

1 Preheat oven to 190°C (375°F/Gas 5). Line 10 x ^{1}/$_3$ cup (80 ml/2^{2}/$_3$ fl oz) muffin holes with muffin cases.
2 Sift the flours and cinnamon into a bowl. Stir in the oat bran, sugar or sweetener, carrot and blueberries and make a well in the centre.
3 Whisk together the egg, buttermilk, apple puree and oil and stir into the dry ingredients until just combined (the mixture should still be lumpy).
4 Divide the mixture among the muffin holes and bake for 20 minutes or until risen and golden.

per muffin (sugar) fat 3.5 g ▌ saturated fat 0.7 g ▌ protein 5.3 g ▌ carbohydrate 26.5 g ▌ fibre 4.2 g ▌ cholesterol 20 mg ▌ sodium 181 mg ▌ energy 703 kJ (168 Cal) ▌ GI low–med ▼–◆

per muffin (sweetener) fat 3.5 g ▌ saturated fat 0.7 g ▌ protein 5.3 g ▌ carbohydrate 24.4 g ▌ fibre 4.2 g ▌ cholesterol 20 mg ▌ sodium 181 mg ▌ energy 669 kJ (160 Cal) ▌ GI low–med ▼–◆

▌ Enjoy in moderation as an occasional treat.

banana & mango smoothies serves 4

1 just-ripe banana, sliced
200 g (6^{1}/$_2$ oz) fresh or
   frozen mango cheeks
50 g (1^{2}/$_3$ oz) dried
   apricots, chopped
1 tablespoon
   unprocessed oat bran

2 cups (500 ml/16 fl oz)
   low-fat milk
1 scoop low-GI low-fat
   vanilla ice cream
2 tablespoons low-fat
   Greek-style plain
   yoghurt

1 Put the banana, mango, apricots, oat bran, milk, ice cream and yoghurt into a blender.
2 Blend thoroughly until thick and smooth. Pour into 4 tall glasses.

per serve fat 0.9 g ▌ saturated fat 0.4 g ▌ protein 7.8 g ▌ carbohydrate 27.7 g ▌ fibre 2.9 g ▌ cholesterol 6 mg ▌ sodium 79 mg ▌ energy 646 kJ (154 Cal) ▌ GI low ▼

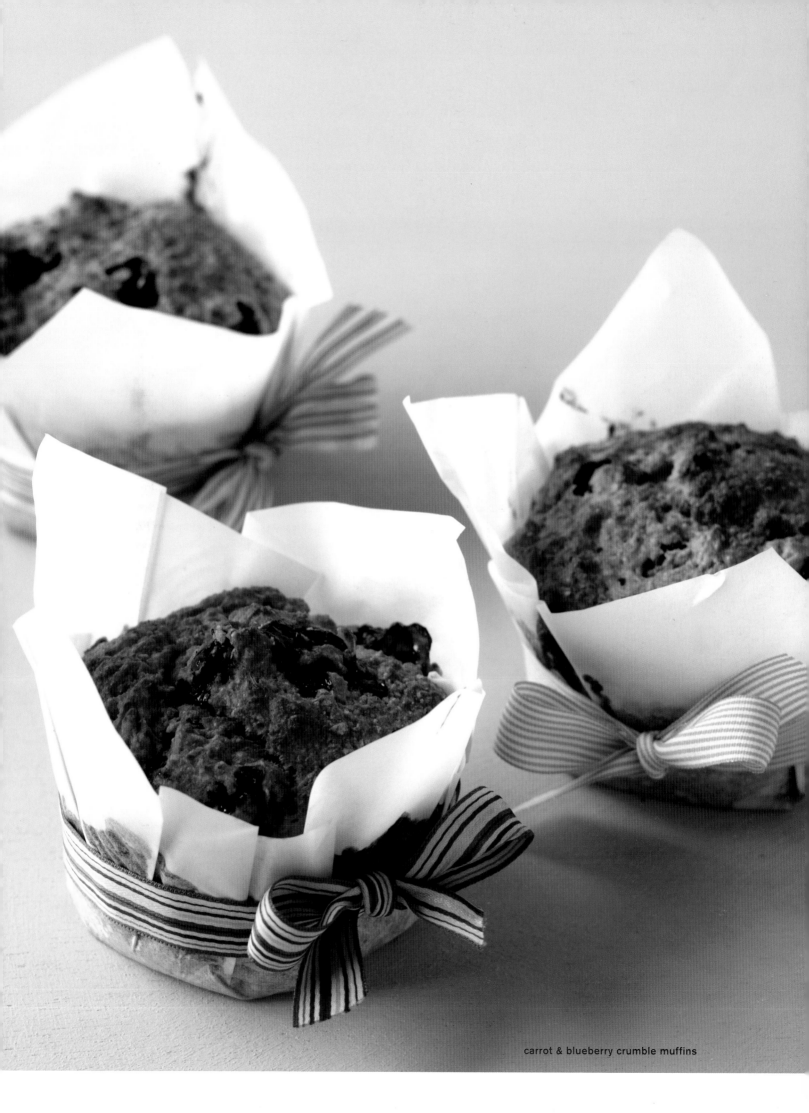

carrot & blueberry crumble muffins

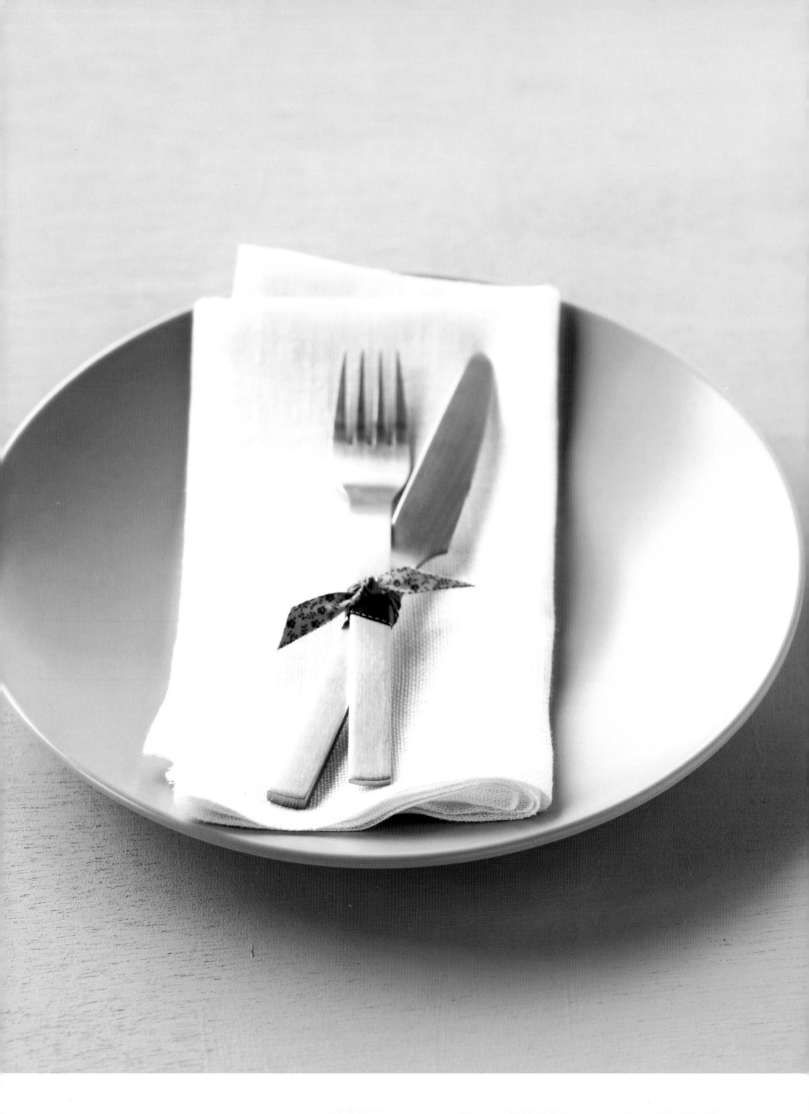

dinner

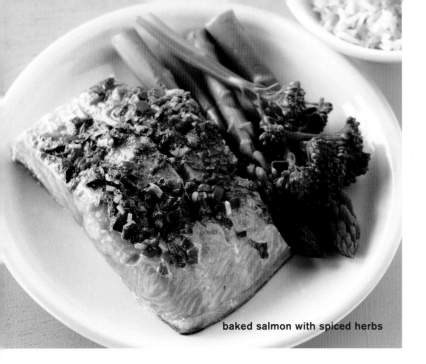
baked salmon with spiced herbs

baked salmon with spiced herbs serves 4

4 (650 g/1 lb 5 oz)
  salmon fillets
2 tablespoons lemon
  juice
1 red chilli, seeded and
  finely diced
2 cloves garlic, crushed
1 teaspoon brown sugar
2 tablespoons fresh
  coriander (cilantro),
  chopped

2 tablespoons fresh
  flat-leaf parsley,
  chopped
2 teaspoons ground
  cumin
2 teaspoons ground
  coriander
200 g (6½ oz) broccolini
200 g (6½ oz) trimmed
  asparagus

1 Preheat oven to 200°C (400°F/Gas 6). Line a baking tray with baking paper.
2 Place the salmon fillets, skin-side down, on the prepared tray. Using a sharp knife, make 3 slits on top of the salmon.
3 Put the lemon juice, chilli, garlic, sugar, fresh coriander, parsley, cumin and ground coriander in a small bowl and mix well. Spread the topping over the salmon and bake for 10–15 minutes or until done to your liking.
4 Meanwhile, steam the broccolini and asparagus until tender.
5 Serve the fish with the steamed vegetables and steamed basmati rice.

per serve fat 12.2 g ▌ saturated fat 2.6 g ▌ protein 35.9 g
▌ carbohydrate 2.8 g ▌ fibre 3.8 g ▌ cholesterol 84 mg
▌ sodium 88 mg ▌ energy 1144 kJ (273 Cal) ▌ GI low–med ▽–◆

lamb rack with french green lentils serves 4

2 lean lamb racks with
  6 cutlets (900 g/
  1 lb 13 oz), scored
½ teaspoon cracked
  black pepper
½ bunch (10 g/⅓ oz)
  fresh thyme
½ bunch (10 g/⅓ oz)
  fresh rosemary
2 teaspoons olive oil
1 onion, chopped
2 cloves garlic, crushed
1 tablespoon fresh
  rosemary, chopped
1½ cups (285 g/9 oz)
  lentils du puy or
  green lentils

2½ cups (625 ml/
  20 fl oz) reduced-salt
  chicken stock
2½ cups (625 ml/
  20 fl oz) water
1 tablespoon wholegrain
  mustard
2 tablespoons balsamic
  vinegar
100 g (3⅓ oz) baby
  English spinach
200 g (6½ oz) green
  beans, trimmed
200 g (6½ oz) broccoli,
  cut into florets

1 Preheat oven to 150°C (300°F/Gas 2).
2 Rub the lamb racks with cracked black pepper. Heat a large heavy-based fry pan over high heat and sear the lamb until well browned.
3 Put the fresh thyme and rosemary sprigs in a baking dish and sit the lamb racks on top. Bake for 25–30 minutes, then remove from the oven, cover and rest for 10–15 minutes.
4 Meanwhile, heat the oil in a large fry pan over medium heat. Add the onion and cook for 10 minutes or until soft. Add the garlic, chopped rosemary and lentils and cook for 2 minutes. Pour in the stock and water and bring to the boil. Reduce the heat, cover and simmer for 35 minutes or until the lentils are soft. Add the mustard, vinegar and spinach and cook for 5 minutes.
5 Meanwhile, steam the beans and broccoli florets until tender.
6 Cut each lamb rack in half and serve on a bed of lentils with the beans and broccoli.

per serve fat 16 g ▌ saturated fat 6.3 g ▌ protein 52.5 g
▌ carbohydrate 32.8 g ▌ fibre 15.4 g ▌ cholesterol 93 mg
▌ sodium 554 mg ▌ energy 2141 kJ (511 Cal) ▌ GI low ▽

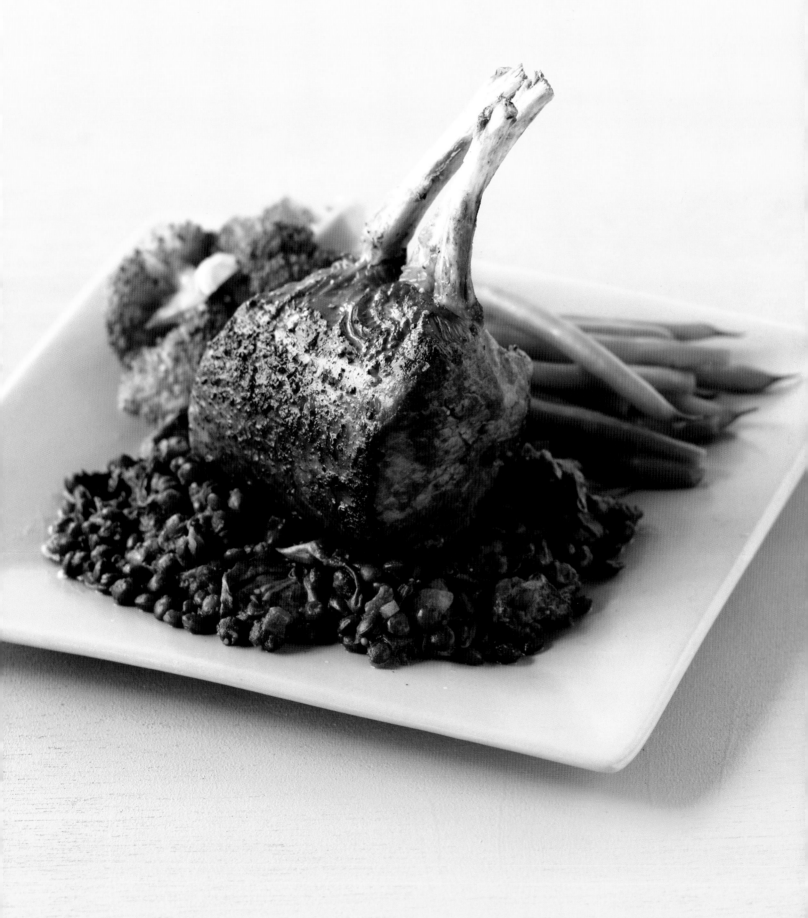

lamb rack with french green lentils

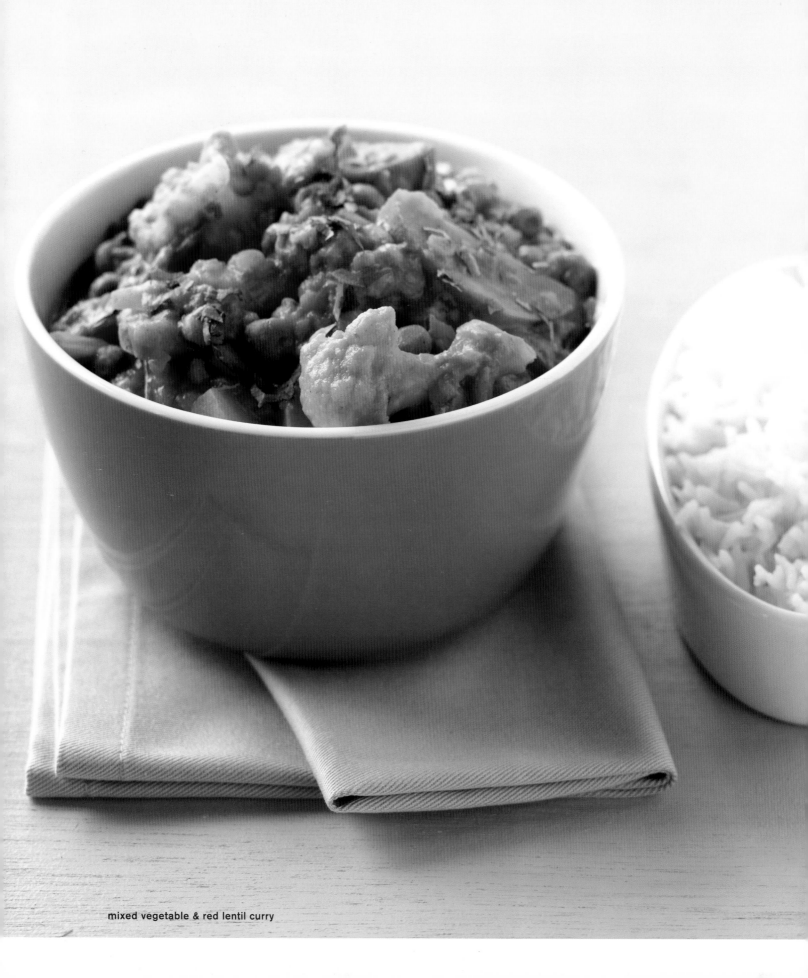

mixed vegetable & red lentil curry

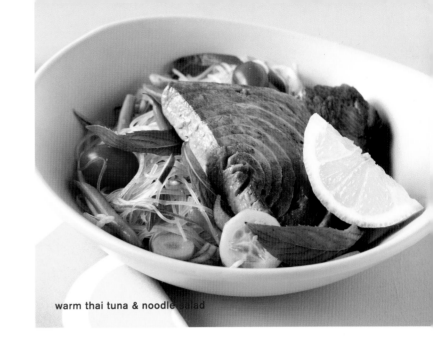
warm thai tuna & noodle salad

mixed vegetable & red lentil curry serves 4

2 teaspoons olive oil
1 onion, chopped
2 cloves garlic, crushed
1 tablespoon grated
   fresh ginger
8 fresh curry leaves
1 teaspoon garam
   masala
1 teaspoon ground
   coriander
1 teaspoon ground
   turmeric
1/2 teaspoon chilli
   powder
1 carrot, chopped
2 new potatoes,
   chopped

300 g (10 oz) orange
   sweet potato, peeled
   and chopped
200 g (6^1/$_2$ oz)
   cauliflower florets
800 g (1 lb 10 oz) can
   chopped tomatoes
2 cups (500 ml/16 fl oz)
   water
1 cup (190 g/6^1/$_4$ oz) red
   lentils
1 cup (155 g/5 oz) peas
1/2 cup (130 g/4^1/$_2$ oz)
   low-fat Greek-style
   plain yoghurt
2 tablespoons chopped
   fresh coriander
   (cilantro)

1 Heat the oil in a large pan over medium heat. Add the onion, garlic and ginger and cook for 5 minutes or until the onion is soft.
2 Add the curry leaves, garam masala, ground coriander, ground turmeric and chilli powder and cook until fragrant.
3 Add the carrot, potatoes, sweet potato, cauliflower, tomatoes and water and bring to the boil. Stir in the lentils, cover and cook for 20 minutes or until the lentils are soft. Stir a couple of times during cooking to stop the lentils from sticking to the pan.
4 Add the peas and cook for 5 minutes. Remove from the heat and stir in the yoghurt. Sprinkle with the coriander and serve with steamed basmati rice.

per serve fat 4.4 g ▮ saturated fat 0.5 g ▮ protein 21.4 g ▮ carbohydrate 49.4 g ▮ fibre 15.6 g ▮ cholesterol 2 mg ▮ sodium 180 mg ▮ energy 1473 kJ (352 Cal) ▮ GI low ▼

warm thai tuna & noodle salad serves 4

4 tuna steaks
100 g (3^1/$_3$ oz) mung
   bean (glass) noodles
100 g (3^1/$_3$ oz) green
   beans, sliced
1 carrot, peeled and
   sliced
1 Lebanese cucumber,
   peeled and sliced
200 g (6^1/$_2$ oz) grape
   tomatoes
1 small red (Spanish)
   onion, thinly sliced

100 g (3^1/$_3$ oz) bean
   sprouts
1 cup (50 g/1^2/$_3$ oz)
   fresh mint
2 tablespoons fish
   sauce
2 tablespoons rice wine
   vinegar or white
   vinegar
1 teaspoon sugar
1 large red chilli, seeded
   and finely chopped
   (optional)
1/2 teaspoon sesame oil

1 Cook the tuna on a lightly oiled chargrill or barbecue plate until done to your liking.
2 Put the noodles into a bowl, cover with boiling water and set aside for 10 minutes or until soft. Drain well.
3 Steam the beans until bright green and tender. Transfer to a bowl and add the carrot, cucumber, tomatoes, onion, bean sprouts, mint and noodles. Toss to combine.
4 Divide the salad among 4 bowls and top with the tuna. Whisk together the fish sauce, vinegar, sugar, chilli and sesame oil and pour over the tuna.

per serve fat 10 g ▮ saturated fat 3.7 g ▮ protein 43.2 g ▮ carbohydrate 28.3 g ▮ fibre 4 g ▮ cholesterol 57 mg ▮ sodium 1013 mg ▮ energy 1629 kJ (389 Cal) ▮ GI low ▼

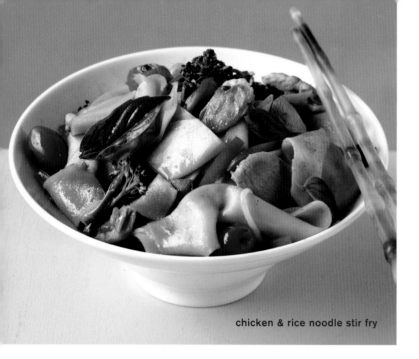

chicken & rice noodle stir fry

chicken & rice noodle stir fry serves 4

2 teaspoons olive oil

300 g (10 oz) skinless
  chicken breast fillet,
  sliced

4 spring onions
  (scallions), sliced

1 red capsicum (bell
  pepper), sliced

200 g (6½ oz) broccolini,
  sliced

200 g (6½ oz) grape
  tomatoes

100 ml (3⅓ fl oz) water

1 tablespoon oyster
  sauce

1 tablespoon fish sauce

1 tablespoon sweet chilli
  sauce

500 g (1 lb) fresh rice
  noodles, cut into
  thick strips

½ cup (15 g/½ oz) Thai
  basil or sweet basil

130 g (4½ oz) bean
  sprouts

1 Heat the oil in a wok over high heat, add the chicken and stir fry until golden brown, then remove.
2 Add the spring onions, capsicum, broccolini, tomatoes and ¼ cup (60 ml/2 fl oz) of the water to the wok and stir fry for 3 minutes or until the vegetables are soft and the water has evaporated.
3 Add the combined oyster sauce, fish sauce, sweet chilli sauce and remaining water and bring to the boil. Stir in the noodles and chicken and toss until heated through.
4 Remove from the heat and fold in the basil and bean sprouts.

per serve fat 4.8 g ▌ saturated fat 0.6 g ▌ protein 27.6 g
▌ carbohydrate 59.2 g ▌ fibre 5.9 g ▌ cholesterol 52 mg
▌ sodium 813 mg ▌ energy 1708 kJ (408 Cal) ▌ GI low ▽

steak with mustard bean mash serves 4

400 g (13 oz) can
  cannellini beans,
  rinsed and drained

400 g (13 oz) can
  chickpeas, rinsed and
  drained

1 onion, grated

1 cup (250 ml/8 fl oz)
  reduced-salt chicken
  stock

2 tablespoons
  wholegrain mustard

1 tablespoon chopped
  fresh rosemary

cracked black pepper

2 teaspoons olive oil

4 lean beef sirloin or eye
  fillet steaks

200 g (6½ oz) button
  mushrooms, sliced

1 cup (250 ml/8 fl oz)
  reduced-salt beef
  stock

1 tablespoon cranberry
  jelly

100 g (3⅓ oz) baby
  English spinach

1 Put the cannellini beans, chickpeas, onion and chicken stock into a pan. Bring to the boil, then reduce the heat and simmer for 10 minutes or until most of the liquid has been absorbed. Remove from the heat. Stir in the mustard, rosemary and cracked black pepper and roughly mash the mixture.
2 Heat the oil in a fry pan over medium heat. Add the steaks and cook for 3 minutes, then turn over and cook the other side until done to your liking. Remove from the pan and keep warm.
3 Add the sliced mushrooms and half the beef stock to the pan and cook for 10 minutes or until the mushrooms are soft and golden. Stir in the remaining stock and cranberry jelly. Bring to the boil and cook over high heat until the sauce has thickened slightly.
4 Wash the spinach and put into a pan. Cover and cook over medium heat for 5 minutes or until wilted. Cool slightly, then squeeze out any excess moisture.
5 Spoon the bean mash onto plates and top with the steaks and mushroom sauce. Serve accompanied with the spinach.

per serve fat 15 g ▌ saturated fat 5.3 g ▌ protein 49 g
▌ carbohydrate 23.3 g ▌ fibre 9.7 g ▌ cholesterol 103 mg
▌ sodium 643 mg ▌ energy 1834 kJ (438 Cal) ▌ GI low ▽

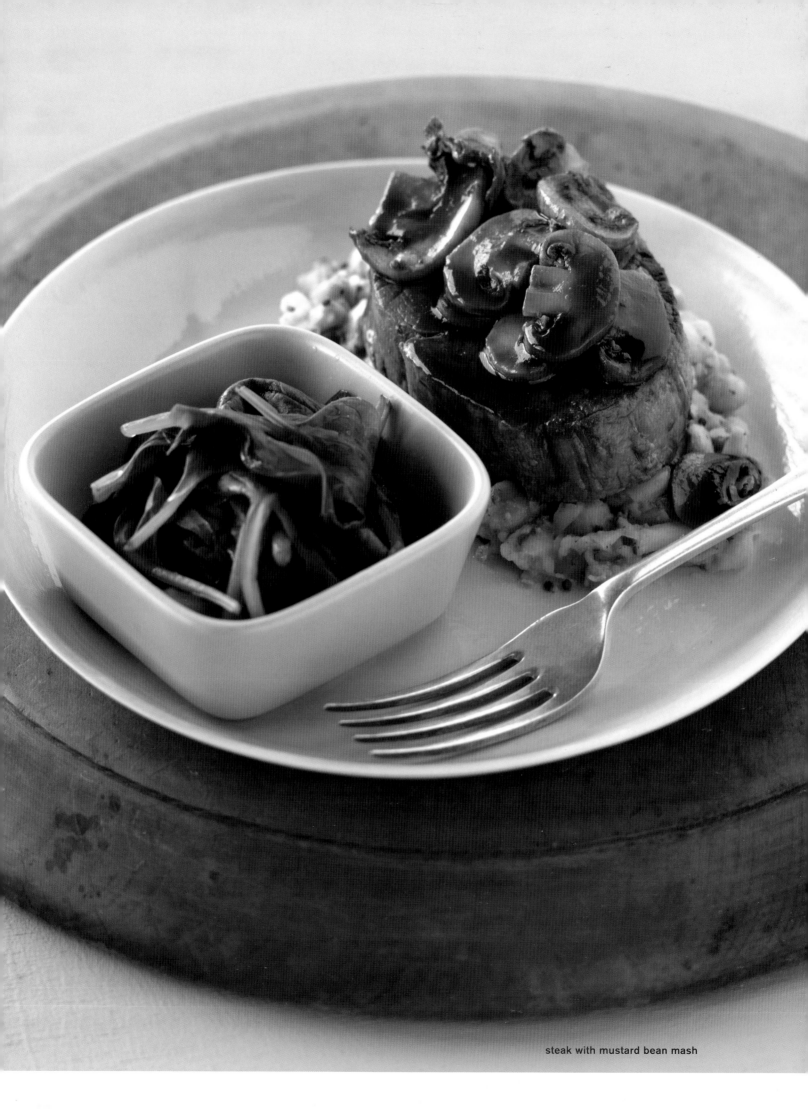

steak with mustard bean mash

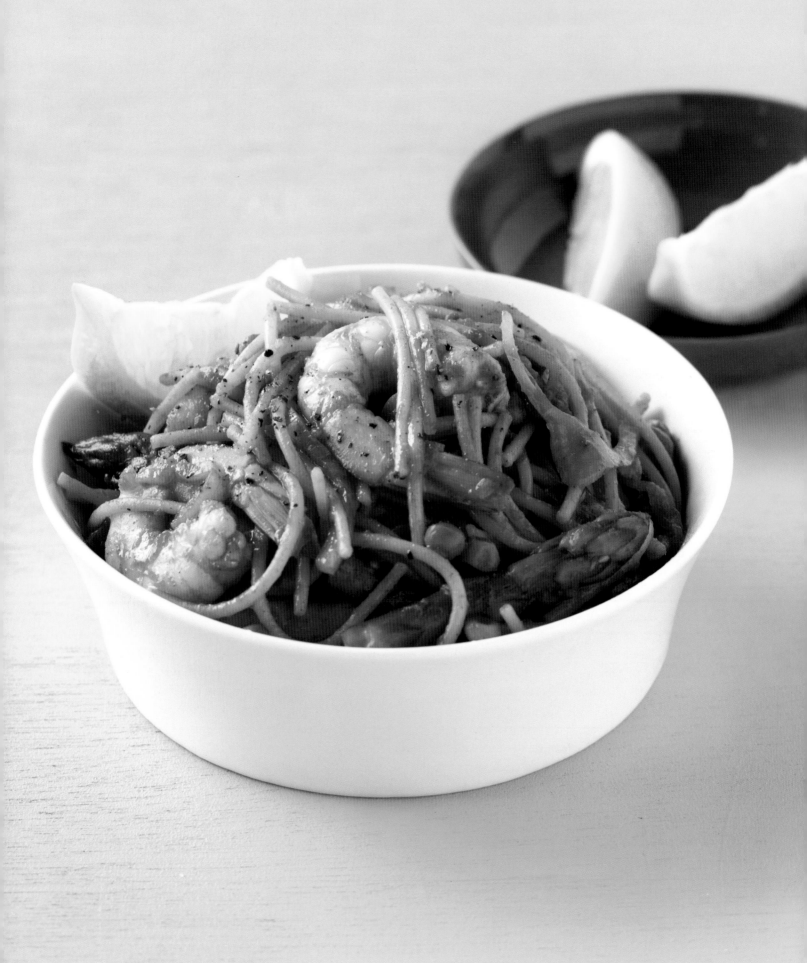

spaghettini with prawns, peas & asparagus

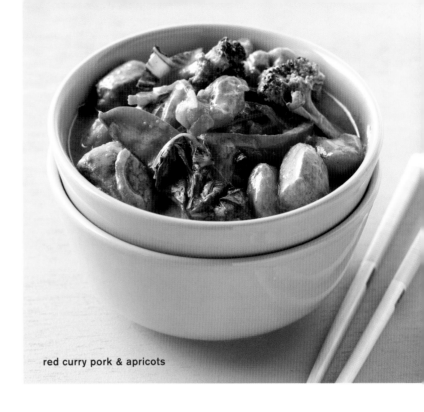

red curry pork & apricots

spaghettini with prawns, peas & asparagus serves 4

1 kg (2 lb) green prawns

1 red (Spanish) onion, chopped

$\frac{1}{2}$ teaspoon saffron threads

2 cups (500 ml/16 fl oz) water

2 teaspoons olive oil

1 fennel bulb, sliced

1 green capsicum (bell pepper), chopped

3 cloves garlic, crushed

1 teaspoon smoked paprika

1 teaspoon sweet paprika

400 g (13 oz) can chopped tomatoes

250 g (8 oz) durum wheat spaghettini, broken into pieces

200 g ($6\frac{1}{2}$ oz) trimmed asparagus, cut into short lengths

1 cup (155 g/5 oz) peas

cracked black pepper

1 Peel and devein the prawns, leaving the tails intact and reserving the shells.

2 Put the prawn shells into a pan and add the onion, saffron and water. Bring to the boil, then reduce the heat and simmer for 10 minutes, skimming off any impurities that rise to the surface during cooking. Strain the stock, discarding the solids. Return the stock to the pan and bring to a simmer.

3 Heat the oil in a large deep fry pan over medium heat. Add the fennel and capsicum and cook for 5 minutes or until the fennel is soft. Add the garlic and paprika and cook for 1 minute or until fragrant.

4 Add the tomatoes, pasta and prawn stock. Bring to the boil and cook for 10 minutes or until the pasta is al dente (cooked, but still with a bite to it).

5 Stir in the prawns, asparagus and peas and cook for 5 minutes or until the prawns are tender. Remove from the heat, cover and set aside for 3 minutes.

6 Sprinkle with cracked black pepper and serve with lemon wedges.

per serve fat 4.6 g ▌ saturated fat 0.6 g ▌ protein 43.6 g ▌ carbohydrate 54.4 g ▌ fibre 9.2 g ▌ cholesterol 223 mg ▌ sodium 616 mg ▌ energy 1911 kJ (456 Cal) ▌ GI low ▽

red curry pork & apricots serves 4

1–2 tablespoons red curry paste

300 g (10 oz) lean pork fillet, cut into 2 cm ($\frac{3}{4}$ in) cubes

1 onion, sliced

1 red capsicum (bell pepper), sliced

2 tablespoons water

100 g ($3\frac{1}{3}$ oz) dried apricots, halved

400 ml (13 fl oz) reduced-fat coconut milk

200 g ($6\frac{1}{2}$ oz) broccoli florets

100 g ($3\frac{1}{3}$ oz) snowpeas

1 bunch (225 g/7 oz) baby bok choy, roughly chopped

1 tablespoon lime juice

1 Heat a wok or fry pan over medium heat. Add the curry paste and cook for 2 minutes or until fragrant.

2 Add the pork and cook for 3 minutes or until browned. Add the onion, capsicum and water and cook until the onion is soft.

3 Stir in the dried apricots and coconut milk. Bring to the boil, then reduce the heat and simmer for 10 minutes. Add the broccoli and snowpeas and cook for 3 minutes or until bright green.

4 Add the bok choy and lime juice and cook for 2 minutes or until the bok choy is soft. Serve with steamed basmati rice.

per serve fat 7.9 g ▌ saturated fat 5.1 g ▌ protein 22.6 g ▌ carbohydrate 20 g ▌ fibre 8.5 g ▌ cholesterol 71 mg ▌ sodium 185 mg ▌ energy 1070 kJ (256 Cal) ▌ GI low ▽

dinner

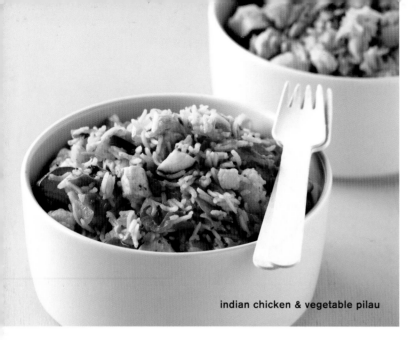
indian chicken & vegetable pilau

indian chicken & vegetable pilau   serves 4

2 teaspoons olive oil
1 teaspoon black
   mustard seeds
1 teaspoon cumin seeds
1 onion, chopped
300 g (10 oz) skinless
   chicken breast fillet,
   chopped
1 green capsicum (bell
   pepper), chopped
200 g (6½ oz)
   cauliflower florets
2 zucchini (courgette),
   chopped

3 tomatoes, chopped
1 cup (200 g/6½ oz)
   basmati rice
½ teaspoon ground
   turmeric
1 cinnamon stick
1½ cups (375 ml/
   12 fl oz) reduced-salt
   chicken stock
1 tablespoon lemon
   juice
3 tablespoons chopped
   fresh coriander
   (cilantro)

1 Heat the oil in a large deep fry pan over medium heat. Add the mustard seeds and cook for 2 minutes or until they start to pop. Add the cumin seeds and cook for 1 minute.

2 Add the onion and cook for 5 minutes or until soft. Stir in the chicken and cook for 5 minutes or until browned.

3 Add the vegetables, rice, turmeric, cinnamon, chicken stock and lemon juice. Bring to the boil, then reduce the heat, cover and simmer without stirring for 15 minutes or until the rice is soft and all the liquid has been absorbed. Stir in the coriander.

per serve fat 4.6 g ▮ saturated fat 0.7 g ▮ protein 26.7 g
▮ carbohydrate 48.6 g ▮ fibre 4.6 g ▮ cholesterol 54 mg
▮ sodium 289 mg ▮ energy 1489 kJ (356 Cal) ▮ GI low ▼

lamb shank casserole with polenta   serves 4

olive oil spray
4 lean lamb shanks
   (2 kg/4 lb), trimmed
1 onion, grated
¼ teaspoon saffron
   threads
2 tablespoons water
2 carrots, peeled and
   cut into chunks
2 teaspoons sweet
   paprika
1 teaspoon hot paprika
800 g (1 lb 10 oz) can
   chopped tomatoes

800 g (1 lb 10 oz) can
   cannellini beans,
   rinsed and drained
2 tablespoons sultanas
1 tablespoon chopped
   fresh rosemary
2 zucchini (courgette),
   cut into chunks
4 cups (1 litre/32 fl oz)
   water, extra
¾ cup (110 g/3½ oz)
   polenta (cornmeal)
¾ cup (120 g/4 oz)
   semolina
cracked black pepper

1 Lightly spray a flameproof casserole dish or large heavy-based pan with olive oil spray and heat over medium heat. Add the lamb shanks and cook until browned all over. Remove from the pan.

2 Add the onion, saffron threads and water to the pan and cook for 3 minutes or until the onion is soft.

3 Return the lamb shanks to the pan and add the carrots, paprika, tomatoes, cannellini beans, sultanas and rosemary. Bring to the boil, then reduce the heat, cover and simmer for 1 hour.

4 Add the zucchini, cover and cook for a further 30 minutes or until the lamb easily comes away from the bone.

5 Meanwhile, bring the extra water to the boil in a pan. Add the combined polenta and semolina in a steady stream, whisking constantly until they start to thicken. Beat with a wooden spoon until the polenta is thick and smooth. Season with cracked black pepper.

6 Serve the lamb shanks and vegetables on a bed of the creamy polenta.

per serve fat 12.8 g ▮ saturated fat 5.7 g ▮ protein 51 g
▮ carbohydrate 72.2 g ▮ fibre 16.1 g ▮ cholesterol 109 mg
▮ sodium 227 mg ▮ energy 2659 kJ (635 Cal) ▮ GI low ▼

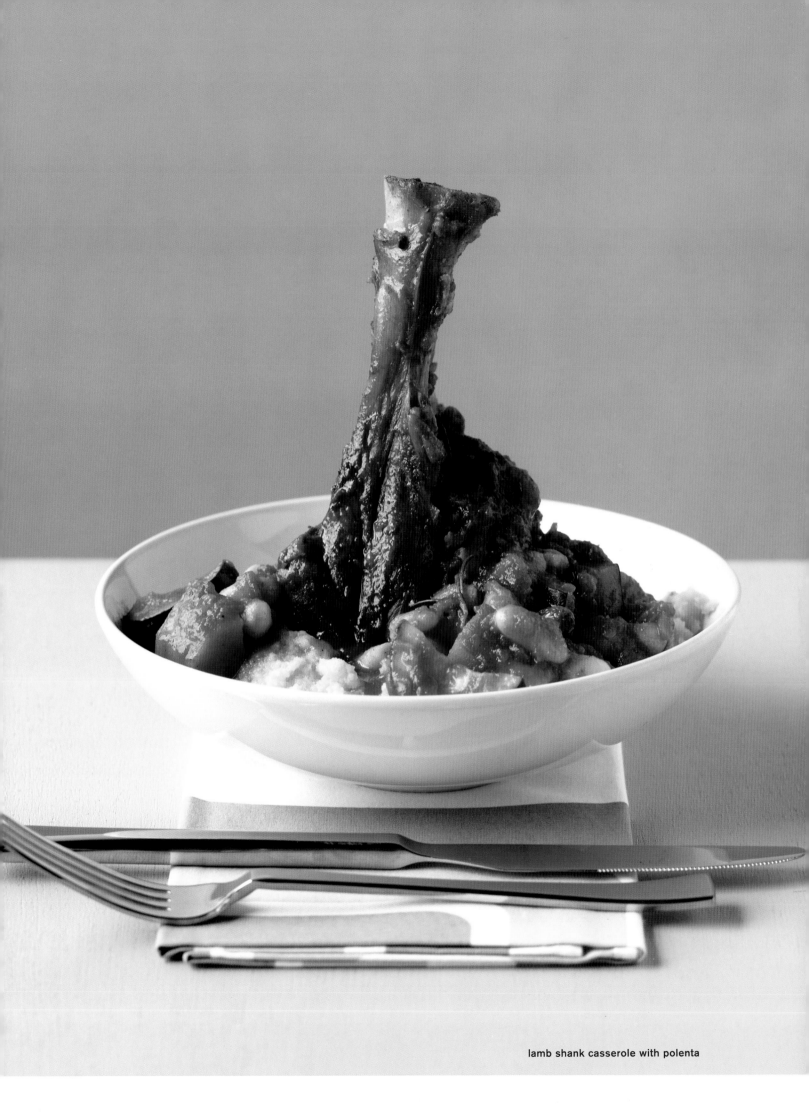

lamb shank casserole with polenta

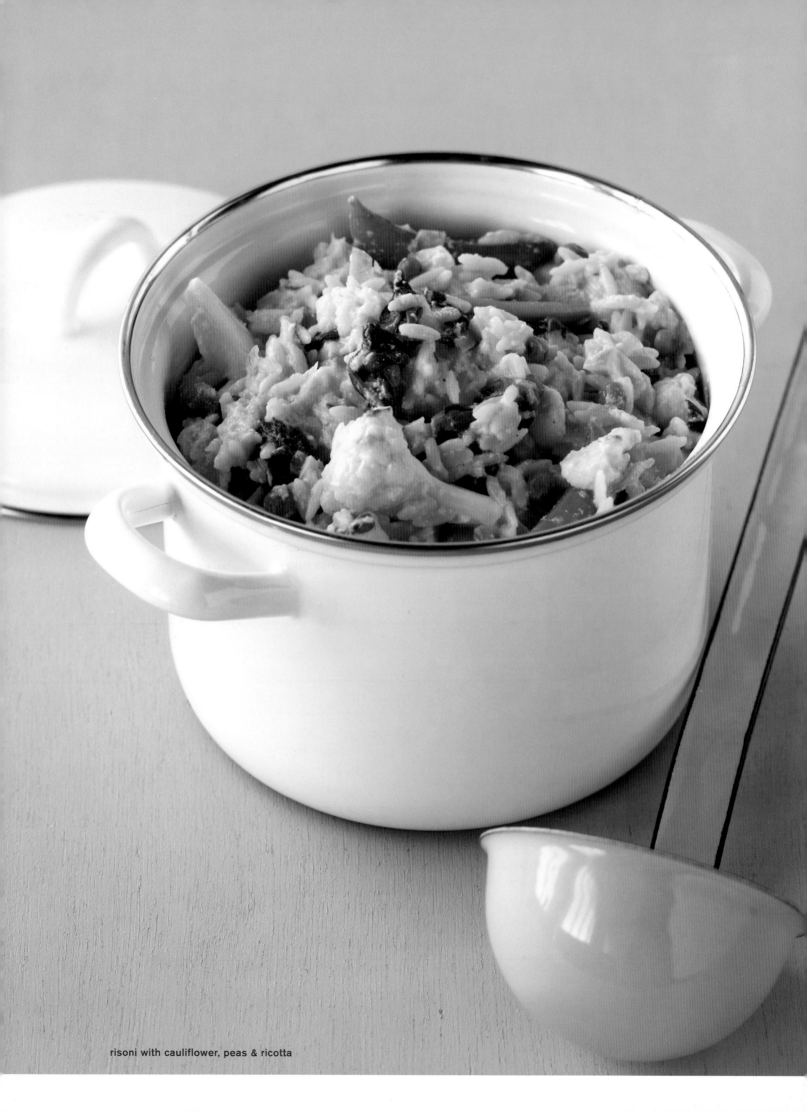

risoni with cauliflower, peas & ricotta

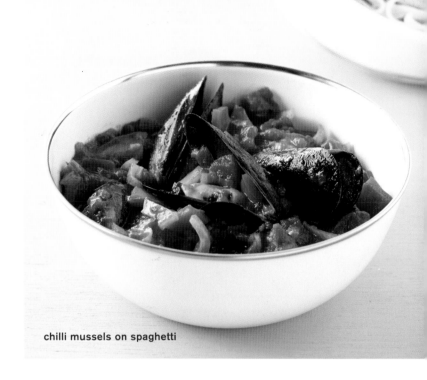

chilli mussels on spaghetti

risoni with cauliflower, peas & ricotta serves 4–6

300 g (10 oz) durum
   wheat risoni
2 teaspoons olive oil
1 onion, chopped
2 cloves garlic, crushed
400 g (13 oz) cauliflower
   florets
1/2 teaspoon saffron
   threads
2 cups (500 ml/16 fl oz)
   reduced-salt chicken
   stock
200 g (61/2 oz) low-fat
   ricotta cheese

1 cup (155 g/5 oz) fresh
   or frozen peas
200 g (61/2 oz) sugar
   snap peas, trimmed
100 g (31/3 oz) baby
   English spinach
2 tablespoons low-fat
   Greek-style plain
   yoghurt
2 tablespoons chopped
   fresh mint
cracked black pepper

1 Cook the risoni in a large pan of rapidly boiling water until al dente (cooked, but still with a bite to it). Drain well.

2 Heat the oil in a large deep fry pan over medium heat. Add the onion and cook for 5 minutes or until golden. Add the garlic and cook for 1 minute.

3 Stir in the cauliflower, saffron and 1/2 cup (125 ml/ 4 fl oz) of the stock and cook for 10 minutes or until the cauliflower is soft.

4 Stir in the risoni, remaining stock, ricotta, peas, sugar snap peas and spinach and cook for 5 minutes or until the vegetables are bright green and tender.

5 Remove from the heat, stir in the yoghurt and mint and season with cracked black pepper. Serve with a vinegar-dressed green salad.

per serve (6) fat 4.3 g ▌ saturated fat 1.1 g ▌ protein 15.1 g ▌ carbohydrate 43.7 g ▌ fibre 6.2 g ▌ cholesterol 2 mg ▌ sodium 272 mg ▌ energy 1213 kJ (290 Cal) ▌ GI low ▼

chilli mussels on spaghetti serves 4

2 teaspoons olive oil
1 onion, chopped
2 cloves garlic, chopped
1 teaspoon chilli flakes
1 red capsicum (bell
   pepper), chopped
1 fennel bulb, thinly
   sliced

800 g (1 lb 10 oz) can
   chopped tomatoes
20 fresh mussels,
   cleaned
2 tablespoons chopped
   fresh parsley
500 g (1 lb) durum
   wheat spaghetti
cracked black pepper

1 Heat the oil in a large pan over medium heat. Add the onion and cook for 5 minutes or until translucent. Add the garlic, chilli flakes, capsicum and fennel and cook for 2 minutes. Stir in the tomatoes, cover and simmer for 25 minutes.

2 Add the mussels and cook over medium heat for 10–15 minutes or until the mussels have opened. Discard any that do not open. Stir in the parsley.

3 Meanwhile, cook the pasta in a large pan of rapidly boiling water until al dente (cooked, but still with a bite to it). Drain well.

4 Divide the spaghetti among 4 bowls and top with the mussels and sauce. Season with cracked black pepper and serve with a vinegar-dressed green salad.

per serve fat 5.8 g ▌ saturated fat 1 g ▌ protein 27.3 g ▌ carbohydrate 100.1 g ▌ fibre 9.3 g ▌ cholesterol 35 mg ▌ sodium 731 mg ▌ energy 2460 kJ (588 Cal) ▌ GI low ▼

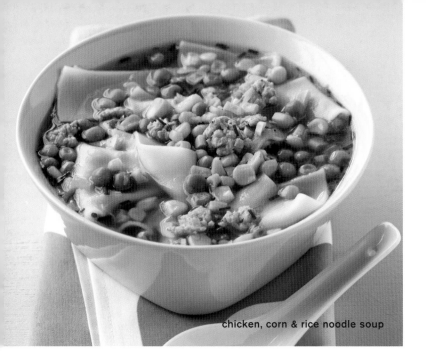

chicken, corn & rice noodle soup

fish with soba & three-chilli dressing serves 4

2 cups (500 ml/16 fl oz) water

4 star anise

8 cardamom pods, crushed

4 firm white fish fillets (snapper)

1 red chilli, seeded and thinly sliced

1 orange chilli, seeded and thinly sliced

1 green chilli, seeded and thinly sliced

1 teaspoon grated palm sugar or brown sugar

2 tablespoons mirin

2 tablespoons lime juice

180 g (6 oz) dried buckwheat soba noodles

2 teaspoons sesame oil

4 baby bok choy, quartered

1 Put the water, star anise and cardamom pods into a large fry pan and bring to the boil. Reduce the heat and simmer for 10 minutes for the flavours to infuse. Add the fish fillets and poach over medium heat for 10–15 minutes or until tender.

2 Put the red, orange and green chillies into a small bowl. Add the sugar, mirin and lime juice and mix until the sugar has dissolved. Set aside to infuse for 10 minutes.

3 Put the noodles into a pan of cold water. Bring to the boil, add another cup of water and stir until boiling. Cook for 5 minutes or until tender. Drain well, transfer to a bowl and toss with the sesame oil.

4 Meanwhile, steam the bok choy until just tender.

5 Serve the noodles with the poached fish, chilli dressing and bok choy.

per serve fat 5.8 g ▮ saturated fat 1.4 g ▮ protein 42.8 g ▮ carbohydrate 35.6 g ▮ fibre 5.1 g ▮ cholesterol 101 mg ▮ sodium 520 mg ▮ energy 1569 kJ (375 Cal) ▮ GI low ▼

▮ Replace the mirin with reduced-salt soy sauce, if preferred.

chicken, corn & rice noodle soup serves 4

2 teaspoons olive oil

1 onion, finely chopped

2 tablespoons grated fresh ginger

200 g (6½ oz) lean chicken mince

½ cup (125 ml/4 fl oz) Chinese rice wine

4 cobs corn, kernels removed

6 cups (1.5 litres/48 fl oz) reduced-salt chicken stock

1½ teaspoons reduced-salt soy sauce

300 g (10 oz) fresh rice noodles, cut into thick strips

1 cup (155 g/5 oz) fresh or frozen peas

2 tablespoons snipped fresh chives

½ teaspoon sesame oil

ground white pepper

1 Heat the oil in a large pan over medium heat. Add the onion and grated ginger and cook for 5 minutes or until the onion is soft.

2 Add the chicken and cook for 5 minutes or until browned. Add the rice wine, bring to the boil and cook over high heat until the liquid is reduced by half.

3 Add the corn, stock and soy sauce, cover and cook for 15 minutes. Add the noodles, peas, chives and sesame oil and cook for 5 minutes or until the noodles and peas are soft. Season with white pepper.

per serve fat 7.7 g ▮ saturated fat 1.4 g ▮ protein 21.6 g ▮ carbohydrate 64.8 g ▮ fibre 9.5 g ▮ cholesterol 46 mg ▮ sodium 1629 mg ▮ energy 1928 kJ (461 Cal) ▮ GI low ▼

▮ Replace the rice wine with extra stock, if preferred.

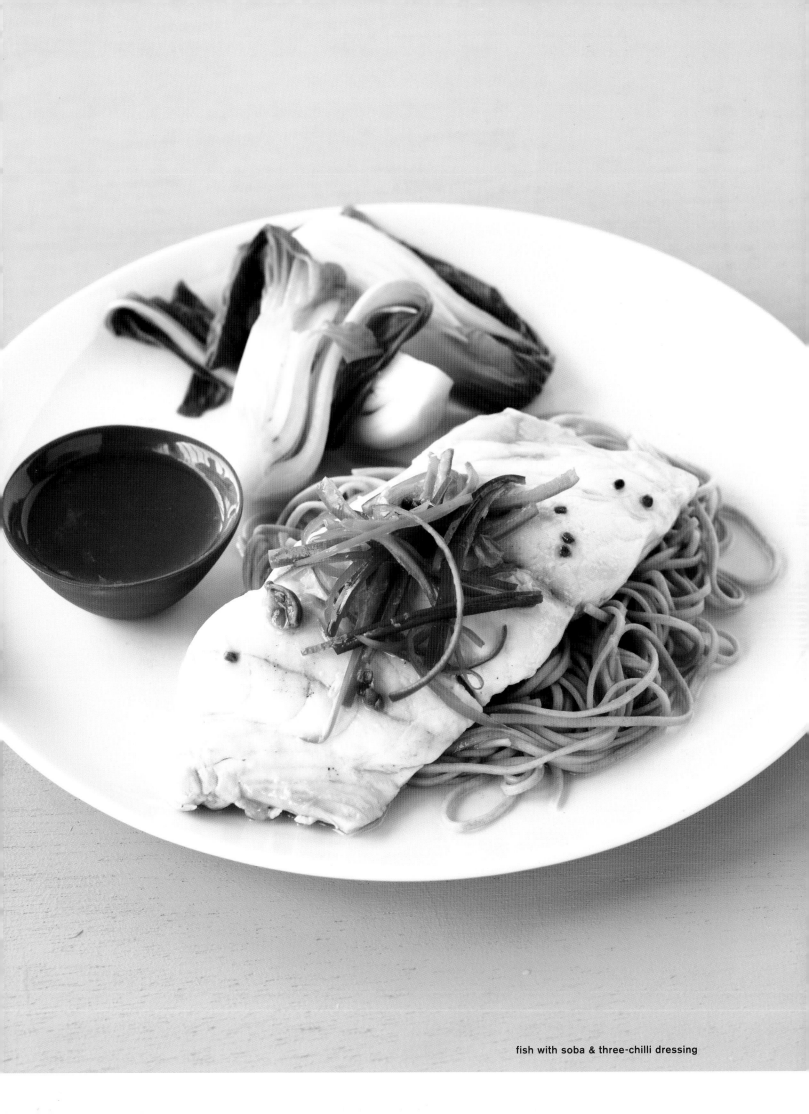

fish with soba & three-chilli dressing

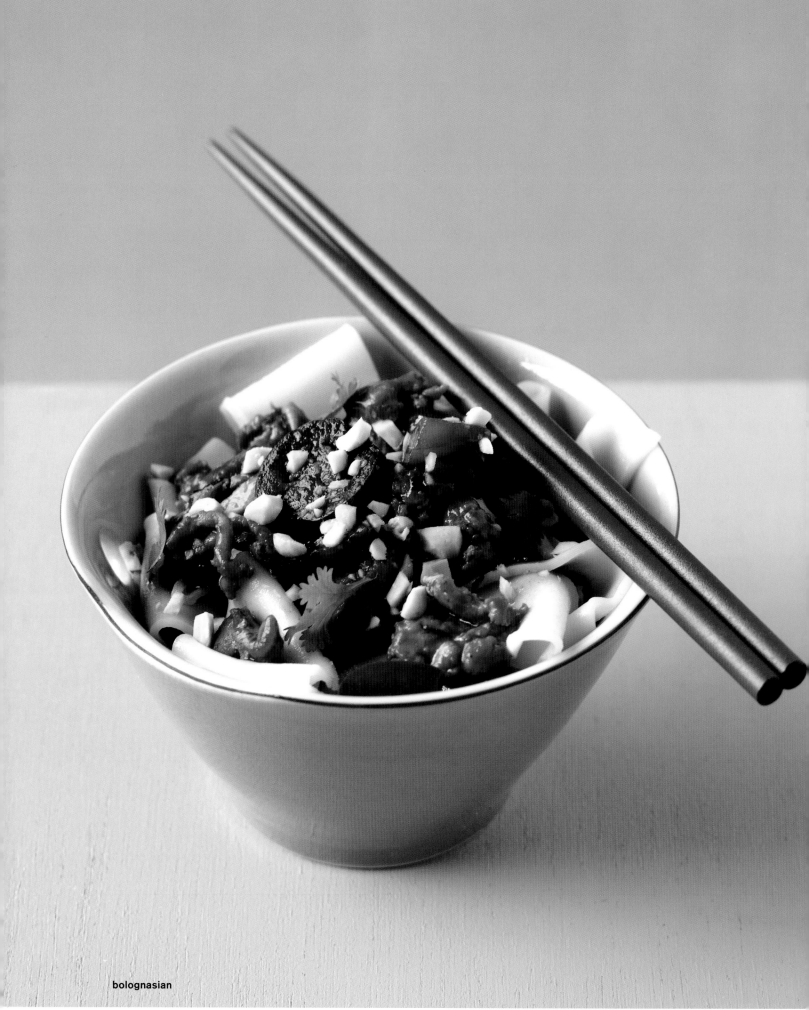

bolognasian

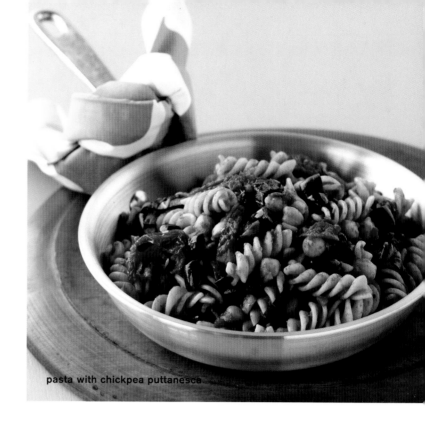

pasta with chickpea puttanesca

bolognasian serves 4

500 g (1 lb) fresh rice
   noodles, cut into
   thick strips
2 teaspoons olive oil
300 g (10 oz) lean pork
   mince
4 spring onions
   (scallions), chopped
1/2 teaspoon minced chilli
100 g (3 1/3 oz) shiitake
   mushrooms, sliced
1 green capsicum (bell
   pepper), chopped
1 Japanese eggplant
   (aubergine), sliced

2 tablespoons kecap
   manis
2 tablespoons tomato
   puree
2 cups (500 ml/16 fl oz)
   reduced-salt chicken
   stock
1 tablespoon cornflour
2 tablespoons water
2 tablespoons chopped
   peanuts
2 tablespoons fresh
   coriander (cilantro)

1 Put the noodles into a bowl, cover with boiling water and set aside for 3 minutes or until soft; drain.
2 Heat the oil in a large fry pan over high heat, add the pork mince and cook for 5 minutes or until browned. Add the spring onions and chilli and cook for 2 minutes.
3 Add the mushrooms, capsicum and eggplant and cook for 5 minutes or until the eggplant is soft.
4 Stir in the kecap manis, tomato puree and stock and bring to the boil. Blend the cornflour with the water and stir into the sauce. Cook, stirring, until the sauce boils and thickens slightly.
5 Serve the sauce on the noodles, sprinkled with the peanuts and coriander.

per serve fat 11.4 g ▮ saturated fat 2.7 g ▮ protein 24.9 g ▮ carbohydrate 60.7 g ▮ fibre 3.9 g ▮ cholesterol 47 mg ▮ sodium 643 mg ▮ energy 1902 kJ (454 Cal) ▮ GI low ▼

pasta with chickpea puttanesca serves 4

350 g (12 oz) durum
   wheat spiral pasta
400 g (13 oz) can
   chopped tomatoes
1/2 teaspoon chilli flakes
100 g (3 1/3 oz) low-fat
   semi-dried tomatoes,
   chopped
100 g (3 1/3 oz) pitted
   kalamata olives,
   chopped

3 tablespoons chopped
   capers
400 g (13 oz) can
   chickpeas, rinsed
   and drained
1 tablespoon red wine
   vinegar
1 teaspoon sugar
3 tablespoons chopped
   fresh basil

1 Cook the pasta in a large pan of rapidly boiling water until al dente (cooked, but still with a bite to it). Drain well.
2 Heat the tomatoes in a large deep fry pan. Add the chilli, semi-dried tomatoes, olives, capers and chickpeas. Bring to the boil, then reduce the heat and simmer for 20 minutes or until the sauce thickens slightly.
3 Stir in the vinegar, sugar and basil. Add the pasta and toss to combine. Serve with a vinegar-dressed green salad.

per serve fat 3.3 g ▮ saturated fat 0.5 g ▮ protein 16.1 g ▮ carbohydrate 83.1 g ▮ fibre 9.3 g ▮ cholesterol 0 mg ▮ sodium 469 mg ▮ energy 1885 kJ (450 Cal) ▮ GI low ▼

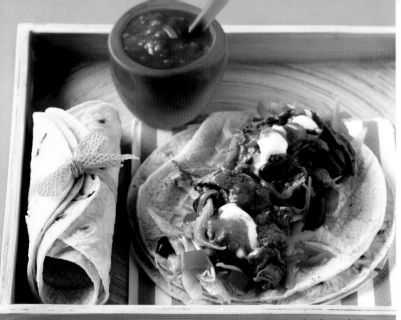
spicy beef & bean fajitas

spicy beef & bean fajitas serves 4

8 medium corn tortillas
2 teaspoons olive oil
300 g (10 oz) lean beef rump steak, thinly sliced
1 red (Spanish) onion, sliced
1/2 teaspoon chilli flakes
1 teaspoon ground cumin
1/2 teaspoon cracked black pepper
300 g (10 oz) can red kidney beans, rinsed and drained
2 tablespoons lime juice
2 cups (115 g/3²/3 oz) shredded lettuce
3 ripe tomatoes, chopped
1 carrot, grated
1/3 cup (85 g/2³/4 oz) low-fat Greek-style plain yoghurt
1 cup (275 g/9 oz) medium tomato salsa

1 Preheat oven to 220°C (425°F/Gas 7). Wrap the tortillas in foil and bake for 10–15 minutes or until heated through.
2 Heat the oil in a large fry pan over high heat. Add the beef and cook for 5 minutes or until browned. Add the onion, chilli, cumin and pepper and cook for 3 minutes or until the onion is soft.
3 Stir in the kidney beans and lime juice and cook for 5 minutes or until the beans are heated through.
4 Serve the warm tortillas topped with the lettuce, tomatoes, carrot, beef mixture, yoghurt and salsa.

per serve fat 7.5 g ▌ saturated fat 2 g ▌ protein 25.9 g ▌ carbohydrate 33.2 g ▌ fibre 9.1 g ▌ cholesterol 49 mg ▌ sodium 613 mg ▌ energy 1369 kJ (327 Cal) ▌ GI low ▼

tofu with ginger & spring onions serves 4

600 g (1 lb 3 oz) silken tofu
2 tablespoons finely shredded fresh ginger
4 spring onions (scallions), shredded
1/2 teaspoon sesame oil
2 teaspoons olive oil
300 g (10 oz) savoy cabbage, sliced
1 bunch (200 g/6¹/2 oz) Chinese broccoli, sliced
2 tablespoons rice wine vinegar
1 tablespoon reduced-salt soy sauce
2 teaspoons yellow box honey

1 Put the tofu on a plate in a large bamboo steamer over a wok of simmering water. Sprinkle the tofu with the ginger and spring onions and drizzle with the sesame oil. Cover and steam for 10 minutes or until the tofu is tender.
2 Meanwhile, heat the olive oil in a wok over high heat. Add the cabbage and stir fry for 3 minutes or until soft. Add the Chinese broccoli and stir fry until wilted.
3 Put the vinegar, soy sauce and honey in a small bowl and mix to combine. Add half the honey mixture to the vegetables and bring to the boil.
4 Cut the tofu into 4 portions and serve drizzled with the remaining honey mixture, accompanied with the vegetables and steamed basmati rice.

per serve fat 13.3 g ▌ saturated fat 1.9 g ▌ protein 20.2 g ▌ carbohydrate 8.5 g ▌ fibre 6.6 g ▌ cholesterol 0 mg ▌ sodium 222 mg ▌ energy 1035 kJ (247 Cal) ▌ GI low ▼

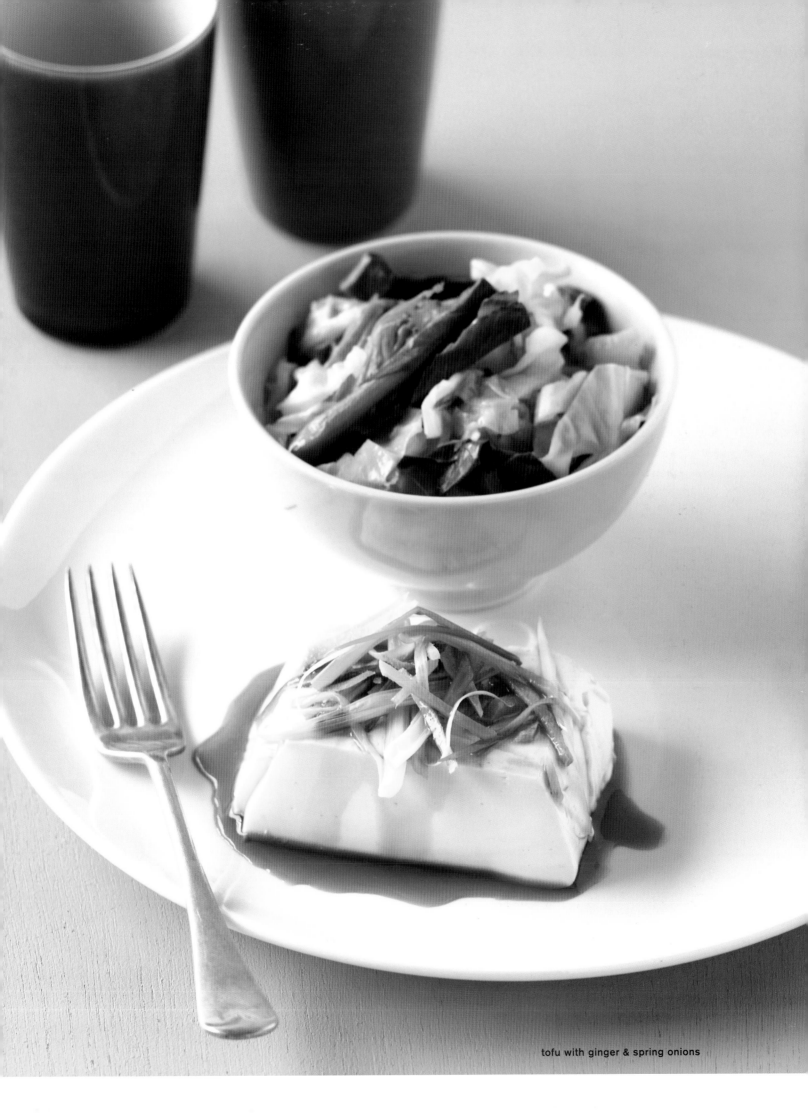

tofu with ginger & spring onions

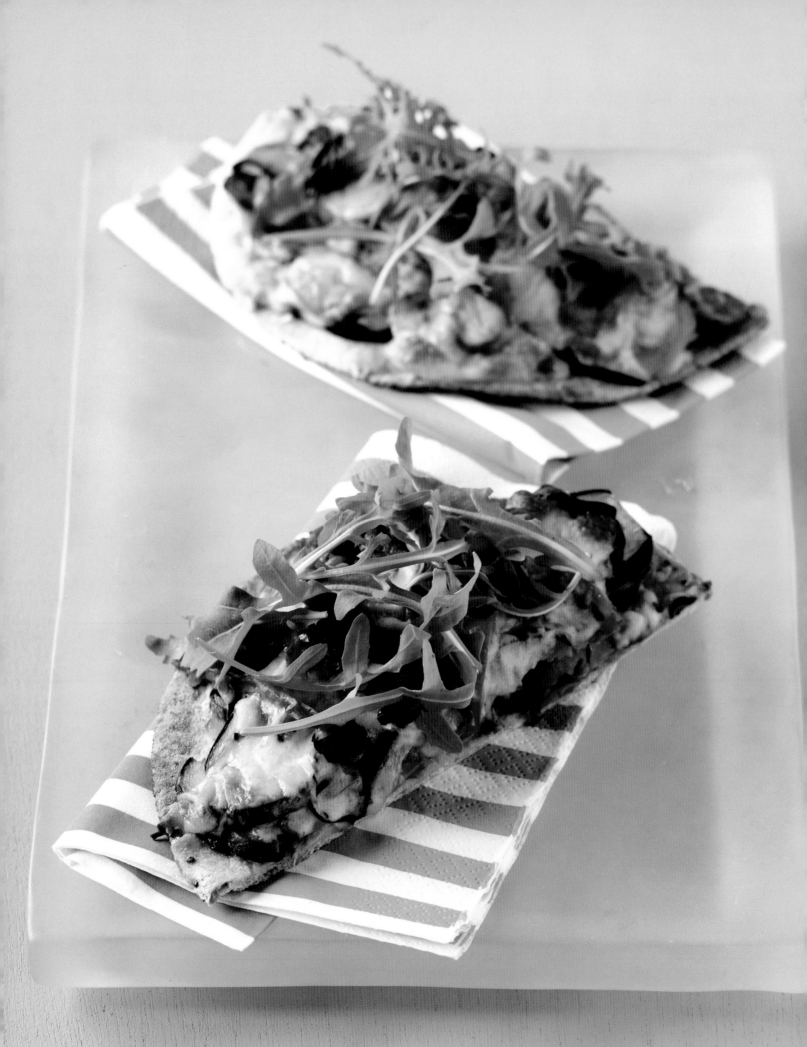

oven-roasted vegetable pizzas

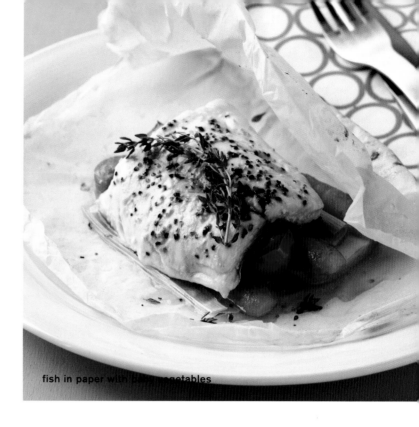

fish in paper with baby vegetables

oven-roasted vegetable pizzas serves 4

200 g (6¹/₂ oz)
mushrooms, sliced

2 zucchini (courgette),
sliced lengthwise

1 small eggplant
(aubergine), sliced

1 red capsicum (bell
pepper), sliced

1 red (Spanish) onion,
chopped

2 cloves garlic, chopped

2 teaspoons olive oil

¹/₄ teaspoon cracked
black pepper

4 small stone-ground
wholemeal pita breads

¹/₃ cup (10 g/¹/₃ oz) fresh
basil

100 g (3¹/₃ oz) low-fat
mozzarella cheese,
grated

30 g (1 oz) rocket
(arugula)

1 Preheat oven to 180°C (350°F/Gas 4).

2 Put the mushrooms, zucchini, eggplant, capsicum, onion, garlic, olive oil and black pepper into a bowl and mix to combine. Spread the mixture on a non-stick baking tray and bake for 20–25 minutes or until the vegetables are soft.

3 Increase the oven to 220°C (425°F/Gas 7). Put the pita breads on a non-stick baking tray. Divide the roasted vegetables, basil and grated mozzarella among the pita breads. Bake for 10 minutes or until the bases are crisp and golden.

4 Scatter the pizzas with the rocket. Serve with a vinegar-dressed green salad.

per serve fat 7.2 g ▌ saturated fat 2.7 g ▌ protein 15.5 g ▌ carbohydrate 30 g ▌ fibre 6.9 g ▌ cholesterol 16 mg ▌ sodium 335 mg ▌ energy 1060 kJ (253 Cal) ▌ GI low ▼

fish in paper with baby vegetables serves 4

1 small leek, thinly sliced

8 baby carrots, halved
lengthwise

4 baby potatoes, sliced

2 spring onions
(scallions), sliced

8 cherry tomatoes,
halved

2 tablespoons verjuice
or lemon juice

4 small boneless
snapper fillets

8 fresh lemon thyme
sprigs

1 tablespoon lemon
juice

2 teaspoons olive oil
cracked black pepper

1 Preheat oven to 220°C (425°F/Gas 7). Cut 4 large heart-shaped pieces of baking paper and fold in half.

2 Put the vegetables and verjuice or lemon juice into a bowl and toss to combine.

3 Arrange the vegetables on one half of each piece of baking paper. Top with the snapper and thyme, drizzle with the combined lemon juice and oil and sprinkle with cracked black pepper. Fold over the paper and put the parcels on a baking tray.

4 Bake the parcels for 15–20 minutes or until puffed and golden.

per serve fat 4.2 g ▌ saturated fat 0.9 g ▌ protein 23.7 g ▌ carbohydrate 17 g ▌ fibre 5.8 g ▌ cholesterol 61 mg ▌ sodium 141 mg ▌ energy 904 kJ (216 Cal) ▌ GI low–med ▼–◆

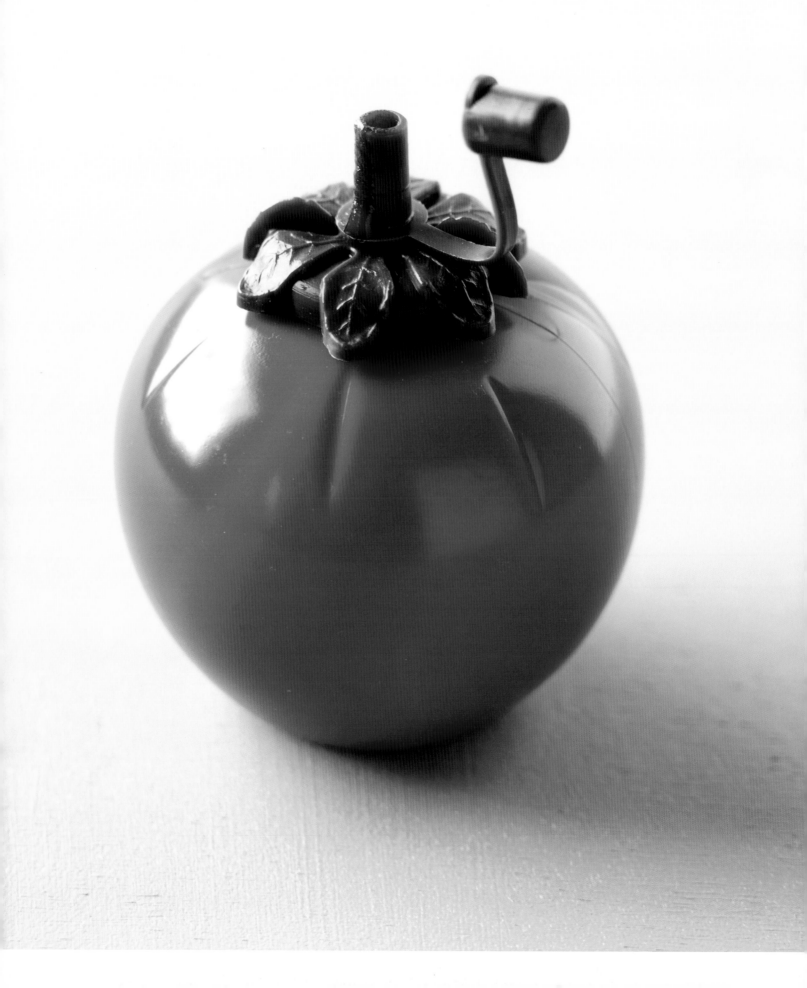

barbecue

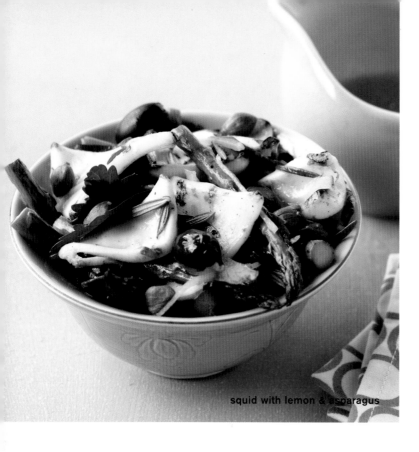

squid with lemon & asparagus

squid with lemon & asparagus serves 4

500 g (1 lb) cleaned baby
  squid tubes, halved
2 bunches (320 g/
  $10^2/_3$ oz) asparagus,
  halved
1 cup (30 g/1 oz)
  chopped fresh flat-leaf
  parsley
2 tablespoons fresh
  rosemary
2 tablespoons pitted
  kalamata olives

1 red (Spanish) onion,
  cut into wedges
2 tablespoons capers
2 cloves garlic, crushed
2 tablespoons lemon
  juice
1 tablespoon white wine
  vinegar
1 tablespoon thinly
  sliced lemon zest
1 tablespoon extra virgin
  olive oil

1 Cook the squid and asparagus on a lightly oiled
barbecue grill until the squid is white and tender
(do not overcook or it will be tough).
2 Put the squid, asparagus, parsley, rosemary,
olives, onion and capers into a bowl. Mix to combine.
3 Whisk together the garlic, lemon juice, vinegar,
lemon zest and olive oil.
4 Drizzle the dressing over the salad. Serve with
wholegrain bread or tabouli.

per serve fat 6.4 g ▌ saturated fat 1.2 g ▌ protein 23.8 g
▌ carbohydrate 6.1 g ▌ fibre 2.7 g ▌ cholesterol 249 mg
▌ sodium 474 mg ▌ energy 778 kJ (186 Cal) ▌ GI low ▼

chunky tofu & vegetable kebabs serves 4

2 zucchini (courgette),
  thickly sliced
1 red capsicum (bell
  pepper), cut into cubes
1 green capsicum (bell
  pepper), cut into cubes
3 spring onions
  (scallions), cut into
  short lengths
100 g ($3^1/_3$ oz) shiitake
  mushrooms

500 g (1 lb) firm tofu,
  cut into cubes
$1/_2$ teaspoon sesame oil
2 tablespoons black rice
  vinegar or malt vinegar
2 tablespoons rice wine
  vinegar
2 tablespoons reduced-
  salt soy sauce
1 tablespoon chopped
  fresh coriander
  (cilantro)

1 Soak 8 bamboo skewers in water for 30 minutes.
2 Thread the zucchini, capsicums, spring onions,
mushrooms and tofu onto the skewers.
3 Cook the skewers on a lightly oiled barbecue grill,
turning several times, until the tofu and vegetables
are golden brown and tender.
4 Whisk together the sesame oil, black rice vinegar,
rice wine vinegar, soy sauce and coriander. Pour the
dressing over the kebabs.

per serve fat 9.4 g ▌ saturated fat 1.3 g ▌ protein 17.9 g
▌ carbohydrate 5.1 g ▌ fibre 4.5 g ▌ cholesterol 0 mg
▌ sodium 386 mg ▌ energy 789 kJ (188 Cal) ▌ GI low ▼

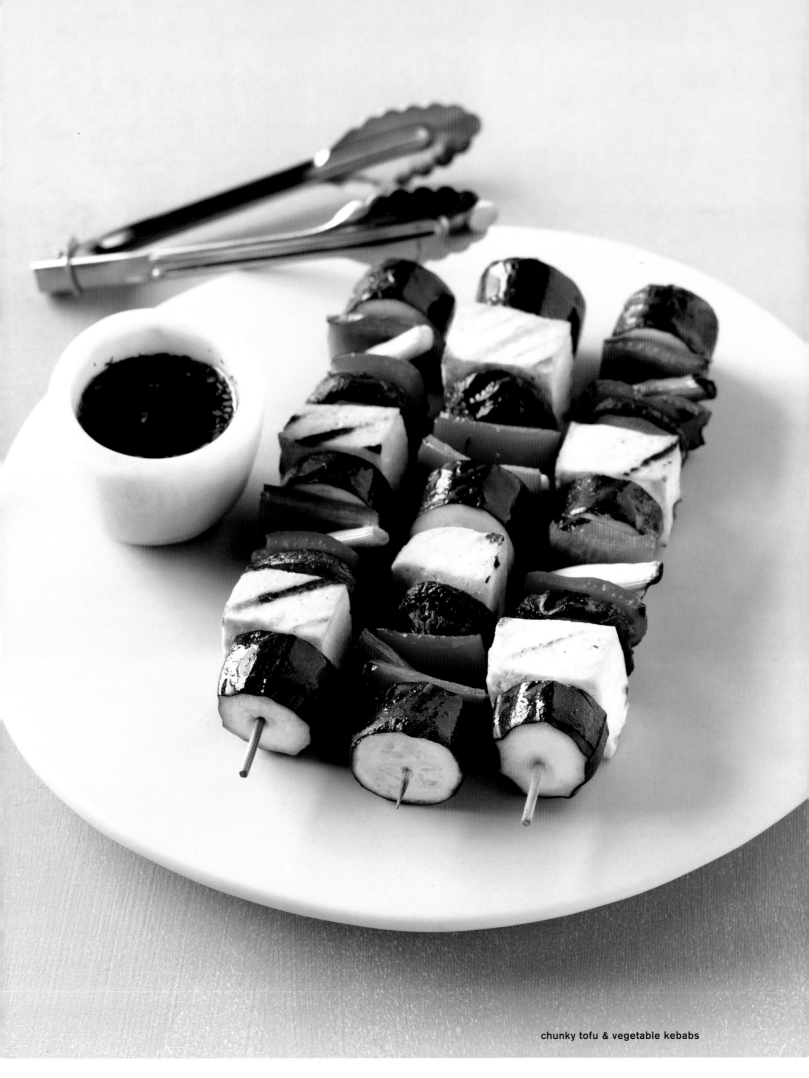

chunky tofu & vegetable kebabs

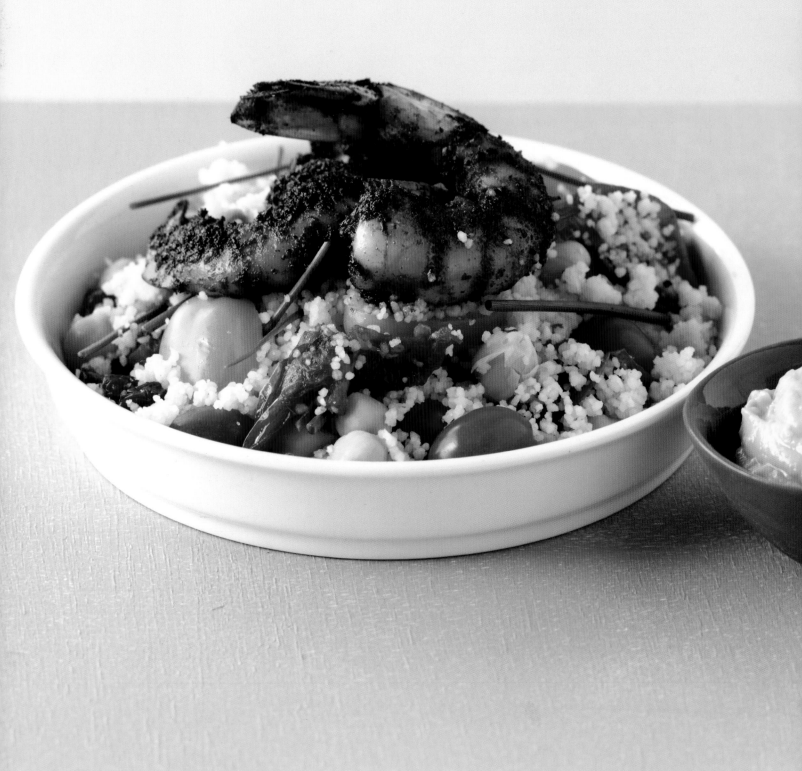

cajun prawns with couscous salad

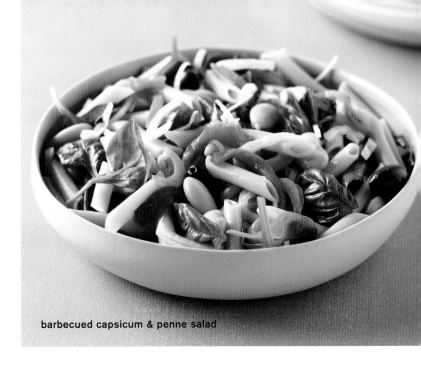

barbecued capsicum & penne salad

cajun prawns with couscous salad serves 6–8

1 tablespoon ground cumin

1 tablespoon ground coriander

1 tablespoon garlic powder

2 tablespoons smoked paprika

2 teaspoons ground white pepper

1/2 teaspoon chilli flakes

1 tablespoon dried Italian herbs

1 kg (2 lb) green prawns, peeled and deveined, tails left intact

1 tablespoon olive oil

1 cup (185 g/6 oz) couscous

1 cup (250 ml/8 fl oz) boiling water

400 g (13 oz) can chickpeas, rinsed and drained

200 g (6 1/2 oz) teardrop tomatoes

200 g (6 1/2 oz) grape tomatoes

100 g (3 1/3 oz) semi-dried tomatoes

2 tablespoons snipped fresh chives

1/2 avocado

1 teaspoon lemon juice

2 tablespoons low-fat Greek-style plain yoghurt

1 Put the spices and dried herbs into a bowl and mix to combine. Add the prawns and toss to coat.

2 Preheat a barbecue flatplate and heat the oil over medium heat. Add the prawns and cook until tender and slightly blackened.

3 Put the couscous into a bowl, pour over the boiling water and set aside for 10 minutes or until the liquid has been absorbed. Separate the couscous grains with a fork.

4 Add the chickpeas, tomatoes and chives to the couscous and gently mix to combine.

5 Mash the avocado in a small bowl. Add the lemon juice and yoghurt and mix to combine.

6 Spoon mounds of the couscous salad onto plates and top with the prawns and a dollop of the avocado mixture. Serve with lemon wedges.

per serve (8) fat 7.8 g ▮ saturated fat 1.3 g ▮ protein 19.8 g ▮ carbohydrate 26.5 g ▮ fibre 5 g ▮ cholesterol 93 mg ▮ sodium 313 mg ▮ energy 1112 kJ (266 Cal) ▮ GI low ▽

barbecued capsicum & penne salad serves 4

200 g (6 1/2 oz) durum wheat penne pasta

1 red capsicum (bell pepper)

1 orange capsicum (bell pepper)

1 fennel bulb, sliced

1 tablespoon lemon juice

2 teaspoons olive oil

400 g (13 oz) can butter beans, rinsed and drained

50 g (1 2/3 oz) baby English spinach

15 pitted black olives

1/2 cup (15 g/1/2 oz) fresh basil

2 teaspoons Dijon mustard

1/4 cup (60 ml/2 fl oz) fresh orange juice

1 clove garlic, crushed

2 teaspoons red wine vinegar

1 Cook the pasta in a large pan of rapidly boiling water until al dente (cooked, but still with a bite to it). Drain well.

2 Cook the capsicums on a hot barbecue grill until blackened. Set aside to cool in a plastic bag, then peel off the skin and slice the flesh.

3 Put the fennel, lemon juice and olive oil into a bowl and toss to combine. Set aside for 10 minutes.

4 Put the pasta, capsicums, fennel, butter beans, spinach, olives and basil into a bowl.

5 Whisk together the mustard, orange juice, garlic and vinegar. Pour over the salad and toss to combine.

per serve fat 3.4 g ▮ saturated fat 0.5 g ▮ protein 9.1 g ▮ carbohydrate 44.2 g ▮ fibre 5.9 g ▮ cholesterol 0 mg ▮ sodium 148 mg ▮ energy 1081 kJ (258 Cal) ▮ GI low ▽

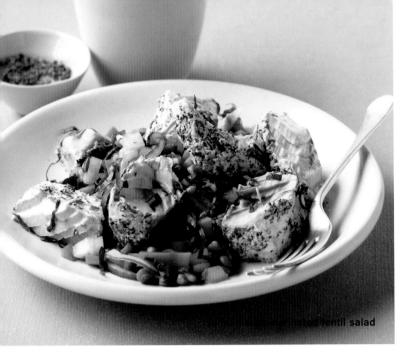

marinated lentil salad

salmon with marinated lentil salad   serves 4

400 g (13 oz) can green
   lentils, rinsed and
   drained
1 carrot, peeled and
   diced
1 Lebanese cucumber,
   unpeeled, diced
1 celery stick, diced
1 red (Spanish) onion,
   sliced
2 tablespoons chopped
   fresh flat-leaf parsley

¼ cup (60 ml/2 fl oz)
   white wine vinegar
1 teaspoon sugar
1 tablespoon cumin
   seeds
1 teaspoon ground black
   pepper
1 tablespoon dried mint
150 g (5 oz) low-fat
   Greek-style plain
   yoghurt
4 salmon steaks

1 Put the lentils, carrot, cucumber, celery, onion and parsley into a non-metallic bowl and mix to combine. Stir in the vinegar and sugar. Cover and marinate overnight.

2 Toast the cumin and pepper in a dry fry pan until fragrant. Transfer to a bowl, add the mint and yoghurt and mix to combine.

3 Rub the yoghurt mixture over the salmon, cover and refrigerate for 2 hours.

4 Wrap the salmon in foil and cook on a preheated barbecue grill or flatplate for 10–15 minutes or until tender. Break into bite-sized pieces and serve with the lentil salad.

per serve fat 11.9 g ▮ saturated fat 2.6 g ▮ protein 37.1 g ▮ carbohydrate 11.5 g ▮ fibre 3.4 g ▮ cholesterol 84 mg ▮ sodium 296 mg ▮ energy 1308 kJ (312 Cal) ▮ GI low ▼

japanese beef with sticky sweet potato   serves 4

¼ cup (60 ml/2 fl oz)
   sake (optional)
1 tablespoon mirin
   (optional)
1 tablespoon yellow
   box honey
¼ cup (60 ml/2 fl oz)
   reduced-salt soy
   sauce
300 g (10 oz) lean beef
   rump steak
300 g (10 oz) orange
   sweet potato, peeled
   and thickly sliced

300 g (10 oz) Japanese
   eggplant (aubergine),
   thickly sliced
olive oil spray
2 tablespoons pickled
   ginger, finely shredded
3 spring onions
   (scallions), sliced
1 mizuna lettuce, leaves
   separated
2 teaspoons black
   sesame seeds
2 teaspoons toasted
   sesame seeds

1 Put the sake, mirin, honey and soy sauce into a pan. Bring to the boil, then cook over high heat for 5 minutes. Set aside to cool completely.

2 Add the beef to the marinade and toss to combine. Refrigerate for 30 minutes.

3 Meanwhile, lightly spray the sweet potato and eggplant with olive oil spray and cook on a preheated barbecue grill for 15–20 minutes or until tender. Arrange on 4 plates and sprinkle with the combined pickled ginger and spring onions.

4 Drain the beef, reserving the marinade, and cook on a preheated barbecue flatplate for 5 minutes or until tender. Set aside for 5 minutes before slicing.

5 Put the reserved marinade into a pan, bring to the boil and cook for 3 minutes.

6 Arrange the beef on top of the vegetables. Drizzle with the marinade and top with the mizuna and sesame seeds.

per serve fat 6.5 g ▮ saturated fat 1.8 g ▮ protein 20.7 g ▮ carbohydrate 19.9 g ▮ fibre 4.5 g ▮ cholesterol 48 mg ▮ sodium 631 mg ▮ energy 1014 kJ (242 Cal) ▮ GI low ▼

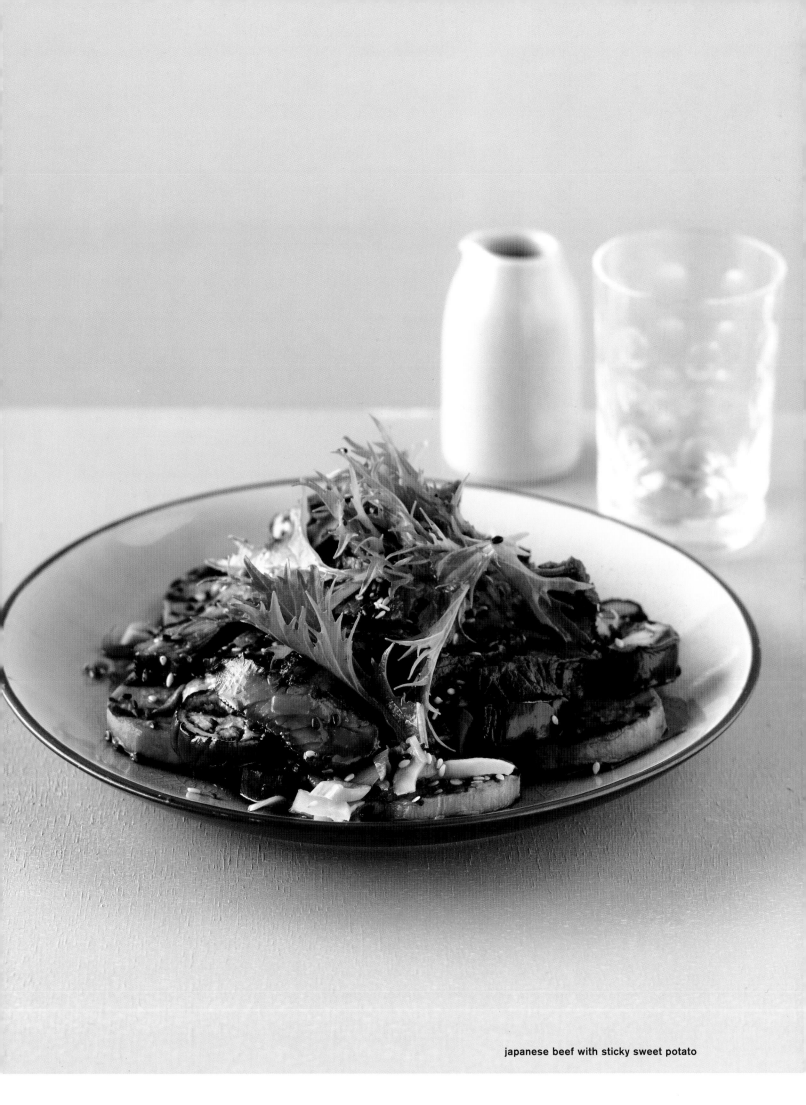

japanese beef with sticky sweet potato

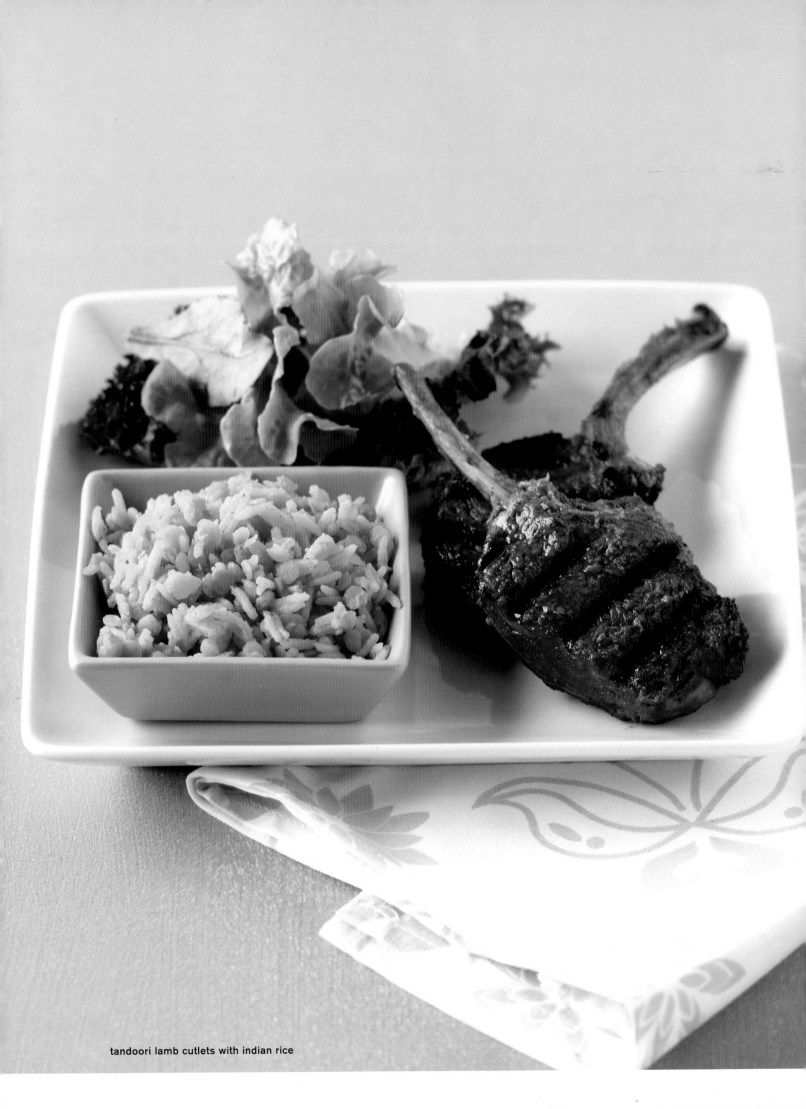

tandoori lamb cutlets with indian rice

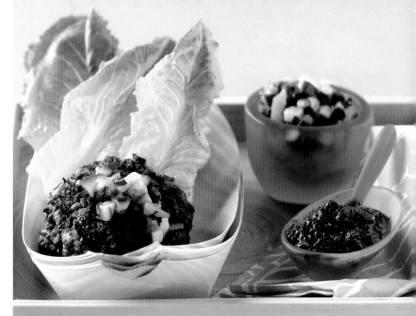

moroccan beef & lentil burgers

tandoori lamb cutlets with indian rice serves 4

200 g (6½ oz) low-fat
   Greek-style plain
   yoghurt
3 tablespoons tandoori
   paste
2 tablespoons grated
   fresh ginger
2 cloves garlic, crushed
8 trimmed lamb cutlets
1 cup (200 g/6½ oz)
   basmati rice
1 cup (190 g/6¼ oz) red
   lentils

1 bay leaf
1 cinnamon stick
2 teaspoons ground
   turmeric
½ teaspoon chilli
   powder
2 cups (500 ml/16 fl oz)
   low-fat mik
1 cup (250 ml/8 fl oz)
   water
2 onions, thinly sliced
2 tablespoons water,
   extra

1 Combine the yoghurt, tandoori paste, ginger and garlic in a non-metallic bowl. Add the lamb and coat evenly in the marinade. Cover and refrigerate for 4 hours or overnight.

2 Put the rice, lentils, bay leaf, cinnamon stick, turmeric, chilli powder, milk and water into a pan and bring to the boil. Cook over high heat until tunnels form in the rice. Reduce the heat to low, cover and cook for 10–15 minutes or until the rice is soft. Discard the bay leaf and cinnamon stick.

3 Cook the lamb cutlets on a preheated barbecue grill over medium heat until tender. Cook the onions with the extra water on a barbecue flatplate until soft and slightly browned.

4 Serve the lamb cutlets and onions with the rice and a little mango chutney.

per serve fat 9.8 g ▮ saturated fat 4.2 g ▮ protein 42.8 g ▮ carbohydrate 76.2 g ▮ fibre 8.2 g ▮ cholesterol 66 mg ▮ sodium 1049 mg ▮ energy 2430 kJ (580 Cal) ▮ GI low ▼

moroccan beef & lentil burgers serves 4

500 g (1 lb) lean beef
   mince
400 g (13 oz) can lentils,
   rinsed and drained
1 onion, grated
50 g (1⅔ oz) pitted
   green olives, chopped
3 large slices wholegrain
   bread, crusts removed,
   torn into small pieces
1 egg white
1 teaspoon ground cumin
1 teaspoon sweet
   paprika

200 g (6½ oz) low-fat
   Greek-style plain
   yoghurt
1 tablespoon finely
   shredded preserved
   lemon
1 Lebanese cucumber,
   unpeeled, finely
   chopped
2 tablespoons finely
   shredded fresh
   parsley
4 wholegrain bread rolls
8 cos lettuce leaves

1 Put the beef, lentils, onion, olives, bread, egg white and spices into a bowl. Using your hands, mix well to combine. Shape the mixture into 8 patties and place on a baking tray lined with baking paper. Cover and refrigerate for 30 minutes.

2 Cook the patties on a lightly oiled barbecue grill until cooked through and golden brown.

3 Combine the yoghurt, preserved lemon, cucumber and parsley and mix to combine.

4 Toast the bread rolls and top with the lettuce, patties and lemon yoghurt. Serve with a little harissa.

per serve fat 12.2 g ▮ saturated fat 4 g ▮ protein 40.3 g ▮ carbohydrate 48.6 g ▮ fibre 7.4 g ▮ cholesterol 67 mg ▮ sodium 807 mg ▮ energy 2026 kJ (484 Cal) ▮ GI low ▼

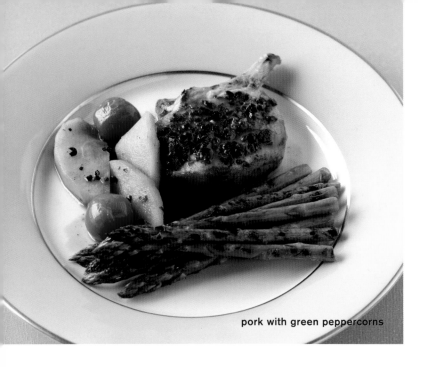

pork with green peppercorns

pork with green peppercorns serves 4

1¹/₂ cups (375 ml/ 12 fl oz) unsweetened low-GI apple juice	3 tablespoons green peppercorns in brine, chopped
2 bay leaves	4 lean pork cutlets
2 large green apples, peeled and cut into eighths	500 g (1 lb) asparagus
	250 g (8 oz) cherry tomatoes
	100 g (3¹/₃ oz) mixed salad leaves

1 Put the apple juice and bay leaves into a pan over high heat and bring to the boil. Add the apples and cook for 10 minutes.
2 Spread half the peppercorns over one side of the pork cutlets. Turn over and sear on a very hot, lightly oiled barbecue flatplate for 5 minutes. Spread the remaining peppercorns on top of the pork, turn and sear for 2 minutes or until tender. Meanwhile, cook the asparagus on the barbecue grill until tender.
3 Drain the apples, reserving the juice. Pour the juice into a heavy-based fry pan and bring to the boil. Add the apples and tomatoes and boil for 5–10 minutes or until the liquid has reduced by half.
4 Serve the pork cutlets with the apples, tomatoes and sauce, accompanied with the asparagus and mixed salad leaves.

per serve fat 4.8 g ▮ saturated fat 1.6 g ▮ protein 23.9 g ▮ carbohydrate 25.8 g ▮ fibre 6.5 g ▮ cholesterol 55 mg ▮ sodium 86 mg ▮ energy 1071 kJ (256 Cal) ▮ GI low ▼

chicken with lime & chilli corn salsa serves 4

4 cobs corn	1 teaspoon sesame oil
2 just-ripe mangoes, chopped	2 cups (170 g/5²/₃ oz) finely shredded Chinese cabbage
3 spring onions (scallions), chopped	1 cup (30 g/1 oz) fresh coriander (cilantro)
6 kaffir lime leaves, finely shredded	¹/₂ cup (15 g/¹/₂ oz) fresh Thai basil
1 large red chilli, shredded	3 tablespoons fresh mint
2 tablespoons lime juice	500 g (1 lb) chicken tenderloins
1 tablespoon fish sauce	

1 Cook the corn on a preheated barbecue grill for 15–20 minutes or until just tender, turning several times during cooking. Set aside to cool slightly.
2 Cut the corn kernels off the cobs and put into a bowl. Add the mangoes, spring onions, lime leaves and chilli and mix to combine.
3 Whisk together the lime juice, fish sauce and sesame oil. Pour over the corn mixture and gently mix to combine.
4 Put the Chinese cabbage, coriander, basil and mint into a large bowl and toss to combine.
5 Cook the chicken on a lightly oiled barbecue grill for 5–10 mintues or until tender.
6 Top the cabbage salad with the chicken and salsa. Serve with lime wedges.

per serve fat 5.3 g ▮ saturated fat 0.8 g ▮ protein 38.9 g ▮ carbohydrate 40.7 g ▮ fibre 10 g ▮ cholesterol 87 mg ▮ sodium 527 mg ▮ energy 1634 kJ (390 Cal) ▮ GI low ▼

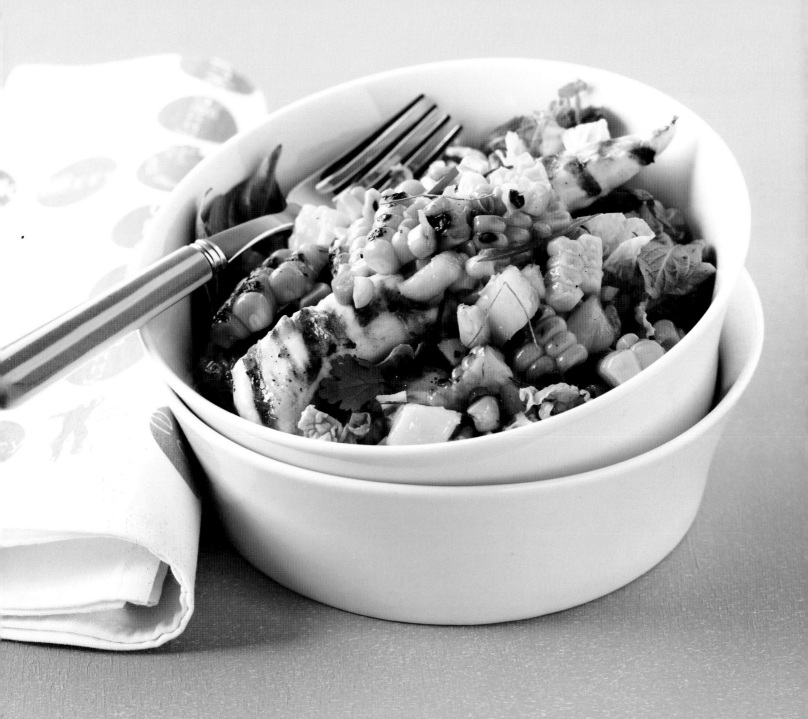

chicken with lime & chilli corn salsa

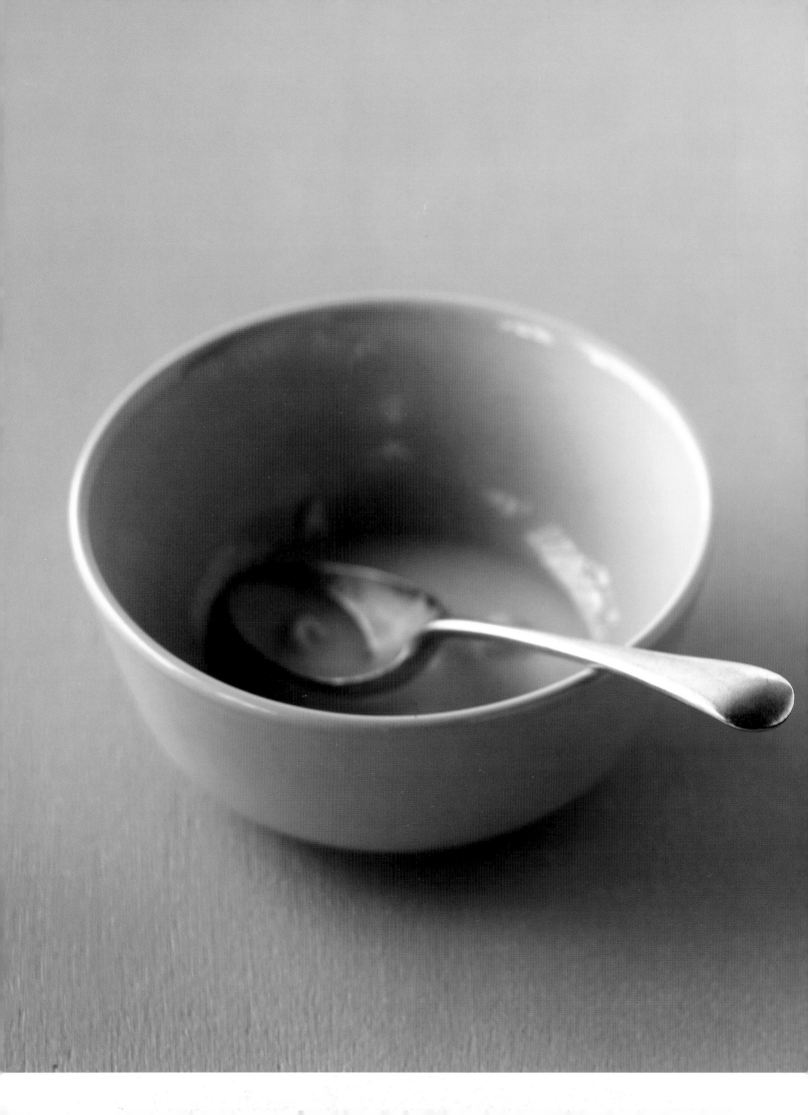

dessert

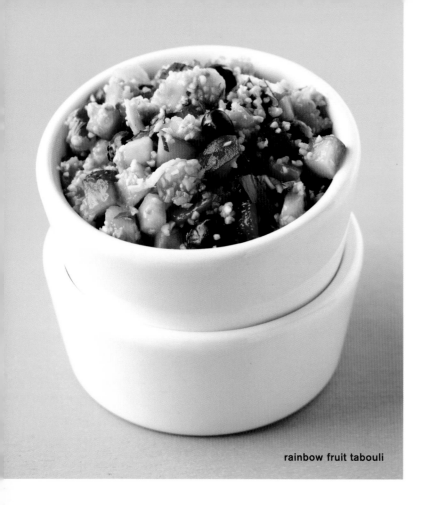

rainbow fruit tabouli

spiced apple crumble serves 4

6 green apples, peeled, cored and cut into wedges

1/2 cup (125 ml/4 fl oz) water

1 teaspoon ground cinnamon

1/2 teaspoon ground ginger

1/4 teaspoon ground black pepper

1/4 teaspoon ground cloves

2 tablespoons caster sugar or low-calorie sweetener suitable for baking

1 cup (100 g/3 1/3 oz) rolled barley

2 tablespoons shredded coconut

1/2 cup (70 g/2 1/4 oz) unprocessed oat bran

2 tablespoons brown sugar or low-calorie sweetener suitable for baking

30 g (1 oz) reduced-fat margarine, melted

1 Preheat oven to 180°C (350°F/Gas 4).

2 Put the apples, water, spices and caster sugar or sweetener into a pan. Cover and cook over medium heat for 10 minutes or until the apples are just soft. Spoon the mixture into an ovenproof dish.

3 Put the rolled barley, coconut, oat bran, brown sugar or sweetener and margarine into a bowl and mix to combine.

4 Sprinkle the topping over the apples and bake for 30 minutes or until the apples are soft and the topping is crisp and golden. Serve with a small scoop of low-GI low-fat vanilla ice cream.

per serve (sugar) fat 7 g ▌ saturated fat 2.5 g ▌ protein 6.1 g ▌ carbohydrate 68.8 g ▌ fibre 10.3 g ▌ cholesterol 0 mg ▌ sodium 7 mg ▌ energy 1516 kJ (362 Cal) ▌ GI low ▼

per serve (sweetener) fat 7 g ▌ saturated fat 2.5 g ▌ protein 6.1 g ▌ carbohydrate 55.9 g ▌ fibre 10.3 g ▌ cholesterol 0 mg ▌ sodium 7 mg ▌ energy 1312 kJ (313 Cal) ▌ GI low ▼

rainbow fruit tabouli serves 4

1/2 cup (70 g/2 1/4 oz) bulgur wheat

1 cup (250 ml/8 fl oz) unsweetened low-GI apple juice

1 tablespoon grated fresh ginger

100 g (3 1/3 oz) strawberries, chopped

100 g (3 1/3 oz) blueberries

2 mangoes, diced

2 peaches, diced

1 cup (50 g/1 2/3 oz) fresh mint, roughly chopped

1 Put the bulgur wheat into a bowl. Pour the apple juice into a pan and add the ginger. Bring to the boil, then pour over the bulgur wheat and set aside for 20 minutes or until the liquid has been absorbed. Transfer to a sieve and press out any excess moisture.

2 Transfer the wheat to a bowl and gently fold in the strawberries, blueberries, mangoes and peaches.

3 Sprinkle with the mint and gently mix to combine. Serve with low-fat Greek-style plain yoghurt.

per serve fat 0.7 g ▌ saturated fat 0.1 g ▌ protein 4.8 g ▌ carbohydrate 38.6 g ▌ fibre 7.7 g ▌ cholesterol 0 mg ▌ sodium 17 mg ▌ energy 832 kJ (199 Cal) ▌ GI low ▼

dessert

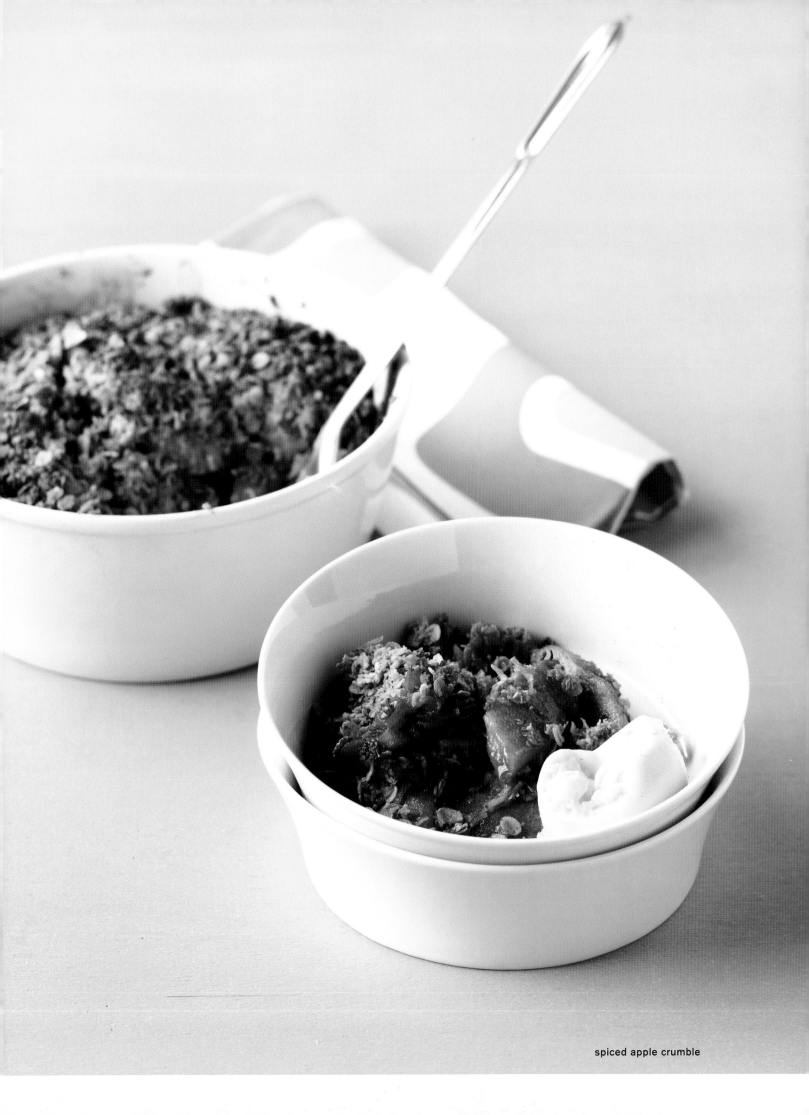

spiced apple crumble

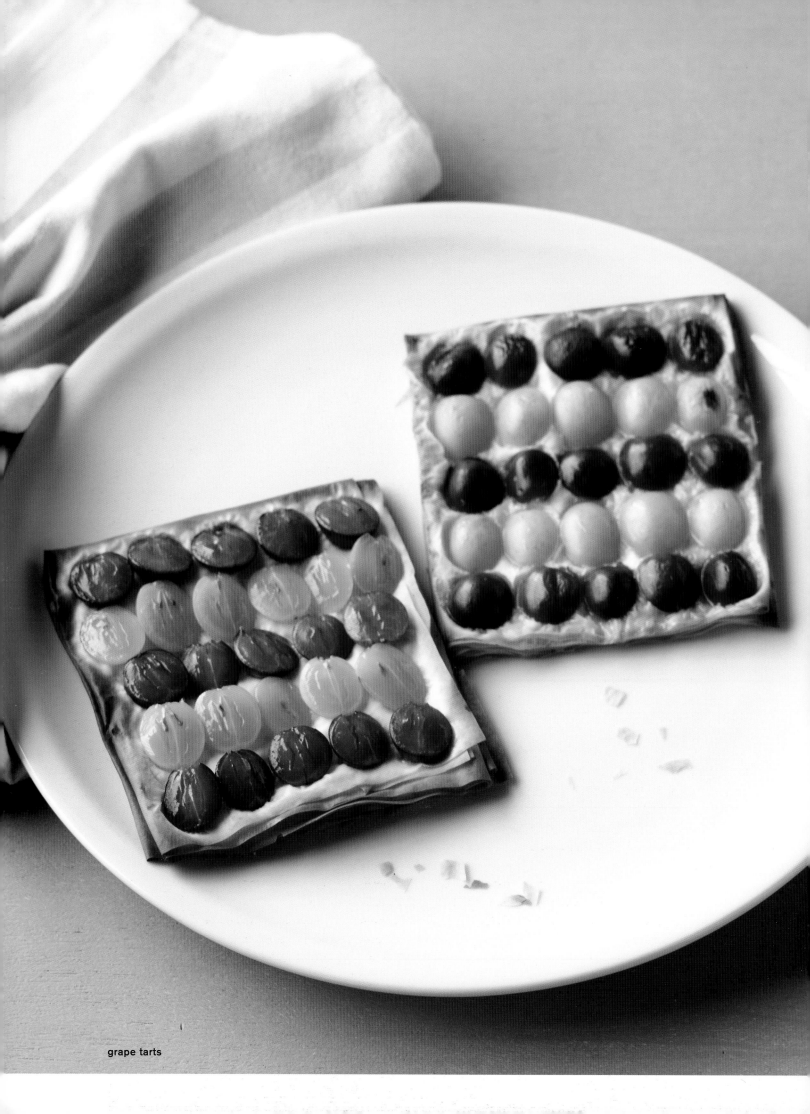

grape tarts

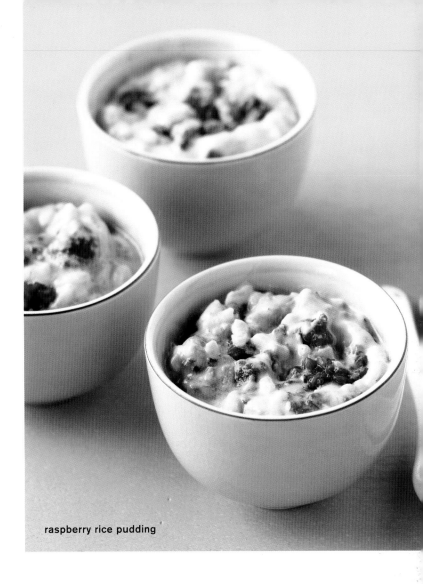
raspberry rice pudding

grape tarts serves 4

8 sheets filo pastry
olive oil spray
120 g (4 oz) seedless
   green grapes, halved
120 g (4 oz) seedless
   red grapes, halved

1 Preheat oven to 220°C (425°F/Gas 7). Line a baking tray with baking paper.

2 Cut each sheet of filo pastry into 4 pieces. Lay 1 piece of pastry on a flat surface. Top with another piece of pastry and lightly spray with olive oil spray. Fold in half and lightly spray again. Repeat with another 6 pieces of pastry. Place on the prepared tray and repeat with the remaining pastry to make 4 tarts.

3 Arrange the grapes in rows over the pastry. Bake for 10 minutes or until the pastry is browned on the edges. Serve with a small scoop of low-GI low-fat vanilla ice cream.

per serve fat 1.8 g ▌ saturated fat 0.3 g ▌ protein 3.1 g ▌ carbohydrate 24.2 g ▌ fibre 1.2 g ▌ cholesterol 0 mg ▌ sodium 202 mg ▌ energy 534 kJ (128 Cal) ▌ GI low–med ▽–◆

raspberry rice pudding serves 4

400 ml (13 fl oz)
   reduced-fat coconut
   milk
2 cups (500 ml/16 fl oz)
   low-fat milk
1 teaspoon vanilla
   essence
120 g (4 oz) koshikari
   short-grain rice
300 g (10 oz) fresh or
   frozen raspberries
1 tablespoon pure maple
   syrup

1 Put the coconut milk, milk and vanilla into a pan and bring to the boil.

2 Add the rice to the pan, reduce the heat and simmer, stirring occasionally, for 25–30 minutes or until the rice is soft.

3 Remove the pan from the heat and stir in the raspberries and maple syrup.

per serve fat 5.6 g ▌ saturated fat 4.6 g ▌ protein 8 g ▌ carbohydrate 43.5 g ▌ fibre 6.4 g ▌ cholesterol 4 mg ▌ sodium 91 mg ▌ energy 1129 kJ (270 Cal) ▌ GI low ▽

dessert

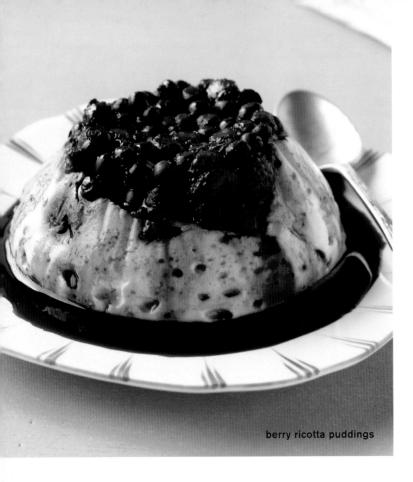

berry ricotta puddings

lime cheesecake with honey pears serves 8

250 g (8 oz) reduced-fat
  ricotta cheese
250 g (8 oz) reduced-fat
  cream cheese
4 tablespoons caster
  sugar or low-calorie
  sweetener suitable
  for baking
2 egg whites, lightly
  beaten
1 teaspoon grated lime
  zest

1 tablespoon lime juice
1 teaspoon vanilla
  extract
3 pears, peeled and cut
  into wedges
1 cup (250 ml/8 fl oz)
  unsweetened low-GI
  apple juice
1 tablespoon yellow box
  honey

berry ricotta puddings serves 4

200 g (6½ oz) fresh or
  frozen mixed berries
500 g (1 lb) fresh low-fat
  ricotta cheese
2 teaspoons rosewater
  (optional)

2 teaspoons yellow box
  honey
2 egg whites, lightly
  beaten

1 Preheat oven to 180°C (350°F/Gas 4). Line the sides of 4 x 1 cup (250 ml/8 fl oz) capacity moulds with baking paper.
2 If using frozen berries, put the berries into a pan with 2 teaspoons of water and gently heat to release the juice. Divide among the prepared moulds.
3 Put the ricotta, rosewater and honey into a bowl and mix well. Fold in the egg whites. Spoon the mixture over the berries.
4 Put the moulds into a baking dish and pour enough boiling water to come halfway up the sides of the moulds. Bake for 15 minutes or until the puddings are set. Invert onto plates and serve.

per serve fat 6.3 g ▌ saturated fat 2.5 g ▌ protein 14.6 g
▌ carbohydrate 10 g ▌ fibre 1.1 g ▌ cholesterol 1 mg
▌ sodium 174 mg ▌ energy 656 kJ (157 Cal) ▌ GI low ▼

1 Preheat oven to 180°C (350°F/Gas 4). Line a 20 cm (8 in) spring form tin with baking paper.
2 Put the ricotta, cream cheese and sugar or sweetener into a bowl. Beat with electric beaters until smooth.
3 Add the egg whites gradually, beating well after each addition. Stir in the lime zest, lime juice and vanilla. Pour the mixture into the prepared tin and bake for 20–30 minutes or until set. Set aside to cool completely, then refrigerate until chilled.
4 Put the pears, apple juice and honey into a fry pan. Cook over medium heat for 10 minutes or until the pears are soft. Remove the pears with a slotted spoon. Bring the liquid to the boil and cook until it has thickened.
5 Cut the cheesecake into slices and serve with the honey pears and syrup.

per serve (sugar) fat 7.9 g ▌ saturated fat 5.2 g ▌ protein 7 g
▌ carbohydrate 24.3 g ▌ fibre 1.1 g ▌ cholesterol 29 mg
▌ sodium 183 mg ▌ energy 818 kJ (195 Cal) ▌ GI low ▼
per serve (sweetener) fat 7.9 g ▌ saturated fat 5.2 g ▌ protein 7 g
▌ carbohydrate 16.8 g ▌ fibre 1.1 g ▌ cholesterol 29 mg
▌ sodium 183 mg ▌ energy 699 kJ (167 Cal) ▌ GI low ▼

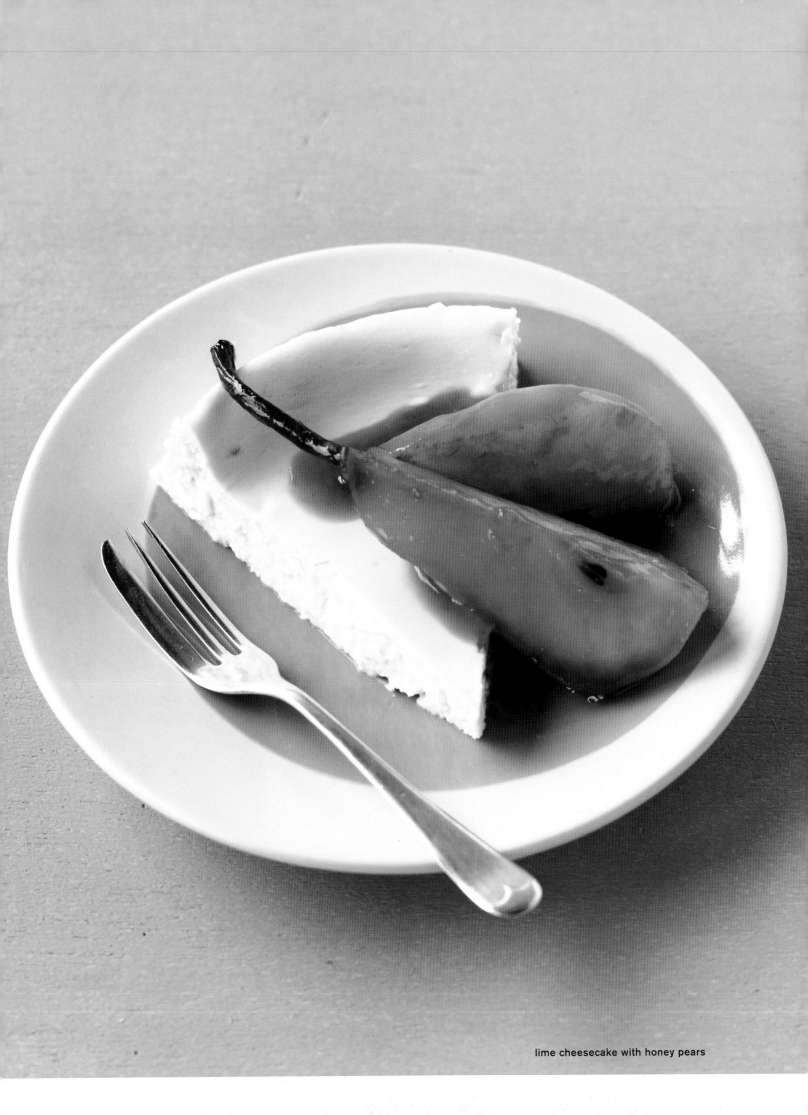

lime cheesecake with honey pears

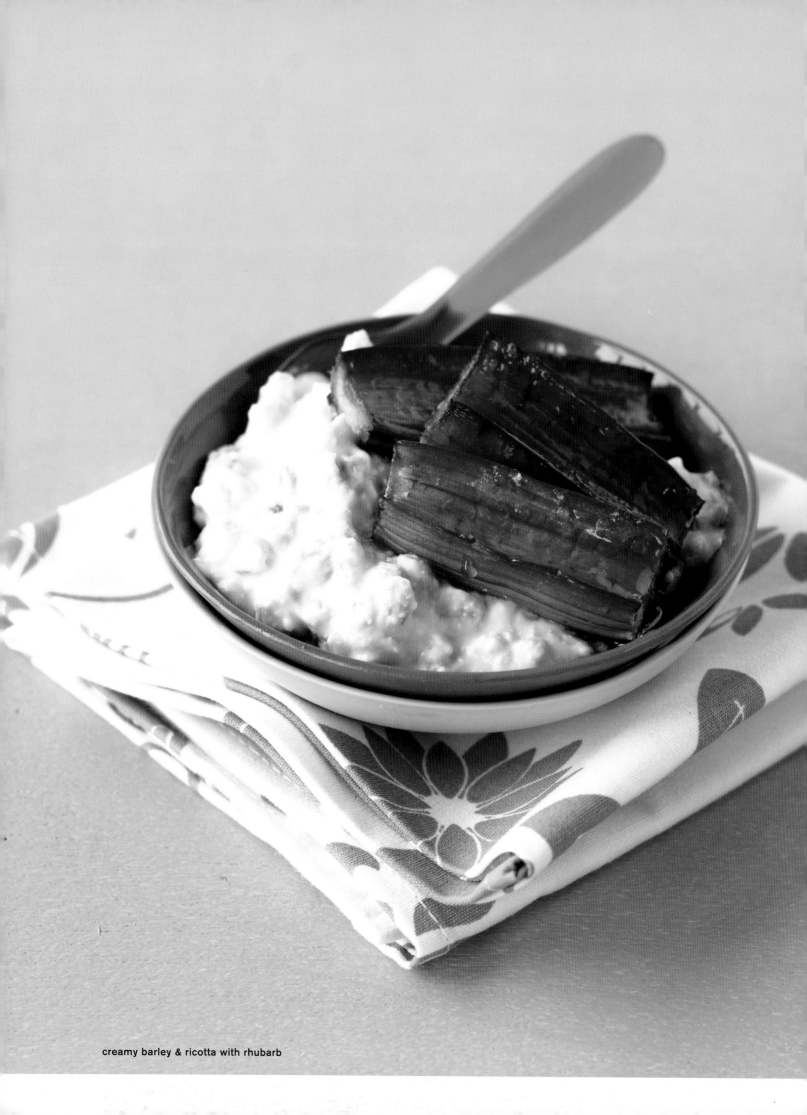

creamy barley & ricotta with rhubarb

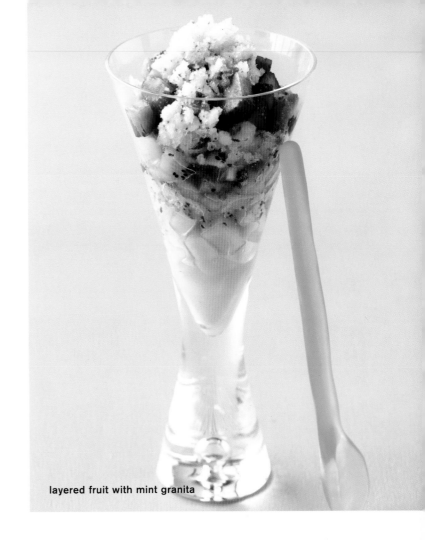

layered fruit with mint granita

creamy barley & ricotta with rhubarb   serves 4

1/2 cup (100 g/3¹/₃ oz)
  pearl barley
250 g (8 oz) low-fat
  ricotta cheese
1 tablespoon yellow box
  honey

1/2 teaspoon almond
  essence
300 g (10 oz) rhubarb,
  cut into short lengths
2 teaspoons sugar or
  low-calorie sweetener
  suitable for baking

1 Preheat oven to 180°C (350°F/Gas 4). Line a baking tray with baking paper.

2 Cook the barley in a large pan of boiling water for 30 minutes or until soft, adding more water if necessary. Rinse under cold water and drain well. Set aside to cool.

3 Put the ricotta, honey and almond essence into a bowl and beat until smooth and creamy. Fold in the cooled barley.

4 Put the rhubarb on the prepared tray, sprinkle with the sugar or sweetener and bake for 15 minutes or until soft.

5 Spoon the creamy barley and ricotta into bowls and top with the baked rhubarb.

per serve (sugar) fat 3.9 g ▌ saturated fat 1.4 g ▌ protein 8.8 g ▌ carbohydrate 28.1 g ▌ fibre 4.2 g ▌ cholesterol 1 mg ▌ sodium 80 mg ▌ energy 803 kJ (192 Cal) ▌ GI low ▼

per serve (sweetener) fat 3.9 g ▌ saturated fat 1.4 g ▌ protein 8.8 g ▌ carbohydrate 26.2 g ▌ fibre 4.2 g ▌ cholesterol 1 mg ▌ sodium 80 mg ▌ energy 773 kJ (185 Cal) ▌ GI low ▼

layered fruit with mint granita   serves 4

3 cups (750 ml/24 fl oz)
  unsweetened low-GI
  apple juice
1 cup (50 g/1²/₃ oz)
  fresh mint, chopped

1 mango, diced
2 kiwifruit, diced
200 g (6¹/₂ oz)
  strawberries, diced

1 Put the apple juice and half the mint into a food processor or blender and blend until smooth. Stir in the remaining mint.

2 Pour the mixture into a shallow non-metallic container and freeze until it starts to harden around the edges. Break up the crystals with a fork and return to the freezer for 1 hour. Repeat the whole process and freeze again.

3 Scrape the granita with a fork and layer into tall chilled glasses with the diced mango, kiwifruit and strawberries.

per serve fat 0.4 g ▌ saturated fat 0 g ▌ protein 2.3 g ▌ carbohydrate 32.1 g ▌ fibre 4.1 g ▌ cholesterol 0 mg ▌ sodium 27 mg ▌ energy 624 kJ (149 Cal) ▌ GI low ▼

dessert

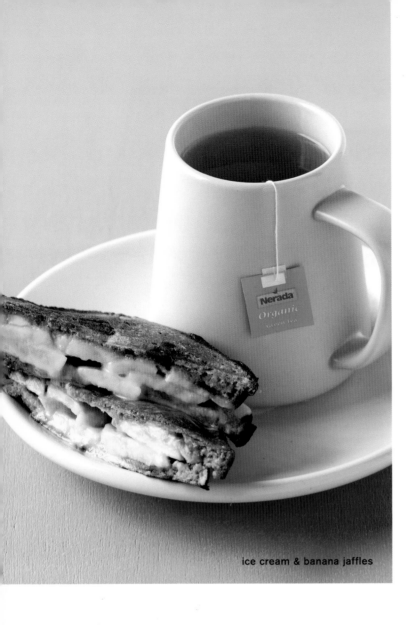

ice cream & banana jaffles

honey yoghurt pots with spiced fruit serves 4

2 teaspoons gelatin

3 cardamom pods, bruised

1¼ cups (310 ml/ 10 fl oz) low-fat milk

1 tablespoon yellow box honey

200 g (6½ oz) low-fat Greek-style plain yoghurt

100 g (3⅓ oz) pitted prunes

100 g (3⅓ oz) dried apricots

1 cinnamon stick

2 teaspoons finely shredded orange zest

1 cup (250 ml/8 fl oz) unsweetened low-GI apple juice

1 Put the gelatin, cardamom pods, milk and honey into a pan. Stir over low–medium heat until the gelatin has dissolved. Set aside to cool.

2 Add the yoghurt to the cooled gelatin mixture and whisk until combined. Strain the mixture into a jug and pour into 4 small cups. Refrigerate for 4 hours or until set.

3 Just before serving, put the prunes, apricots, cinnamon stick, orange zest and apple juice into a pan. Bring to the boil and cook until the fruit is plump and the liquid has thickened slightly. Discard the cinnamon stick.

4 Serve the yoghurt pots with the poached fruit.

per serve fat 0.3 g ▌saturated fat 0.1 g ▌protein 8.9 g ▌carbohydrate 41.7 g ▌fibre 4.3 g ▌cholesterol 5 mg ▌sodium 94 mg ▌energy 893 kJ (213 Cal) ▌GI low ▼

ice cream & banana jaffles serves 4

8 slices spiced dense wholegrain fruit bread

2 small just-ripe bananas, sliced

4 small scoops low-GI low-fat vanilla ice cream, firmly frozen

1 Preheat a non-stick jaffle maker.

2 Arrange half the bread in the jaffle maker. Divide the bananas among the bread and top with the ice cream and remaining bread slices.

3 Cook for 3 minutes or until the bread is crisp and golden. Serve immediately.

per serve fat 2.6 g ▌saturated fat 0.7 g ▌protein 5.3 g ▌carbohydrate 37.4 g ▌fibre 4.2 g ▌cholesterol 2 mg ▌sodium 137 mg ▌energy 844 kJ (202 Cal) ▌GI low ▼

▌Enjoy in moderation as an occasional treat.

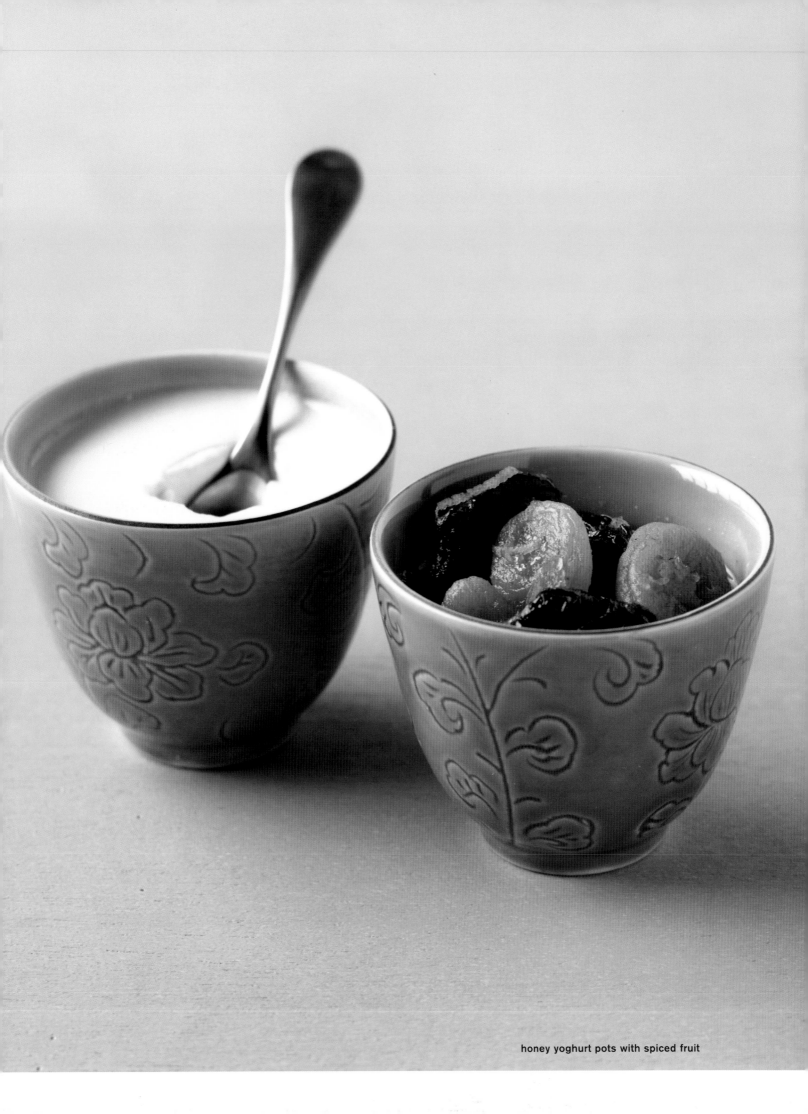

honey yoghurt pots with spiced fruit

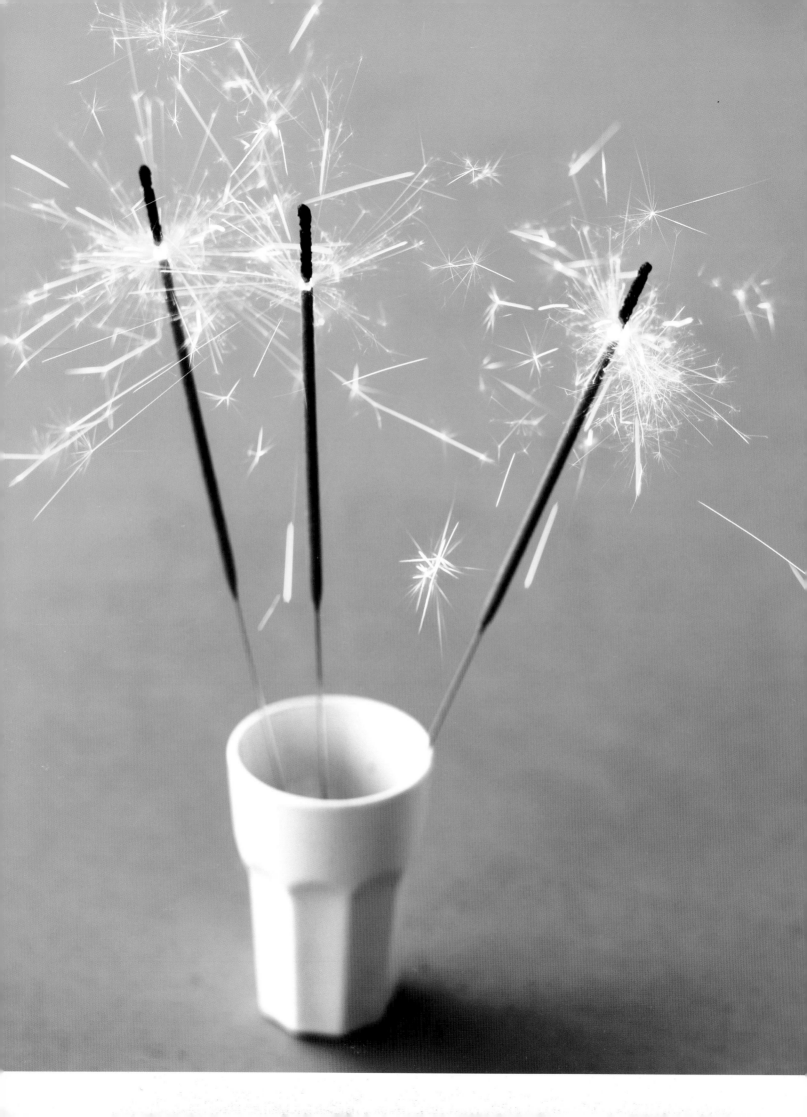

celebration

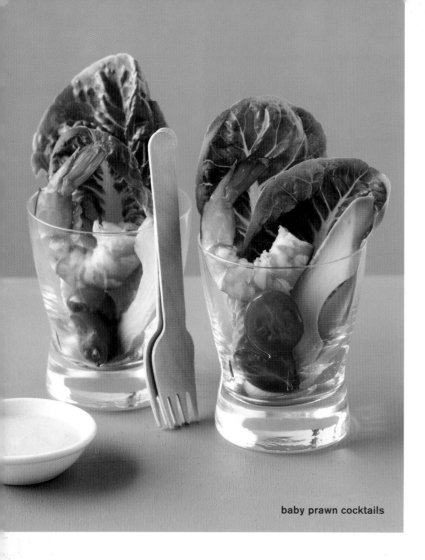
baby prawn cocktails

nori rolls makes 32 pieces

400 g (13 oz) koshikari short-grain rice	½ Lebanese cucumber, peeled and thinly sliced lengthwise
3 cups (750 ml/24 fl oz) water	¼ red capsicum (bell pepper), thinly sliced
120 ml (4 fl oz) rice wine vinegar	1 tablespoon pickled ginger, sliced
4 dried shiitake mushrooms	50 g (1⅔ oz) smoked salmon, sliced
4 sheets nori seaweed	1 teaspoon sesame seeds
1 teaspoon wasabi (optional)	1 teaspoon black sesame seeds
½ small avocado, sliced	

1 Put the rice and water into a large pan. Bring to the boil over high heat and cook until tunnels form in the rice. Remove from the heat and set aside, covered, for 15 minutes or until tender.
2 Transfer the rice to a large bowl and gradually add the vinegar, mixing well with a knife. Set aside to cool.
3 Put the mushrooms into a bowl and cover with boiling water. Set aside for 10 minutes, then drain. Discard the stalks and thinly slice the caps.
4 Lay a sheet of nori on a work surface. Spread the rice over two-thirds of the nori and dot with wasabi. Top with half the avocado, a quarter of the mushrooms, cucumber, capsicum and pickled ginger and roll up to enclose the filling. Repeat to make another roll, replacing the avocado with salmon.
5 Cut 2 sheets of plastic wrap just larger than the nori and spread half the remaining rice into 2 squares the same size as the nori. Lay a sheet of nori on a work surface and dot with wasabi. Top with the remaining avocado and half the mushrooms, cucumber, capsicum and pickled ginger. Roll up to enclose the filling, place on one of the rice squares and roll up in the rice. Remove the plastic and roll in half the combined sesame seeds. Repeat to make another roll, replacing the avocado with salmon.
6 Cut each nori roll into 8 pieces. Serve with reduced-salt soy sauce.

per piece fat 0.6 g ▎ saturated fat 0.1 g ▎ protein 1.4 g ▎ carbohydrate 10.4 g ▎ fibre 0.4 g ▎ cholesterol 1 mg ▎ sodium 37 mg ▎ energy 227 kJ (54 Cal) ▎ GI low ▼

baby prawn cocktails makes 24

48 baby cos lettuce leaves	2 tablespoons low-fat Greek-style plain yoghurt
24 cooked king prawns, peeled and deveined, tails left intact	1 tablespoon low-fat mayonnaise
1 avocado, cut into thin wedges	1 tablespoon lime juice
24 cherry tomatoes, halved	1½ tablespoons tomato sauce

1 Arrange 2 lettuce leaves, a prawn, a wedge of avocado and 2 tomato halves in 24 shot glasses.
2 Whisk together the yoghurt, mayonnaise, lime juice and tomato sauce.
3 Carefully spoon some of the dressing onto each prawn cocktail.

per cocktail fat 2.5 g ▎ saturated fat 0.5 g ▎ protein 4.4 g ▎ carbohydrate 1.3 g ▎ fibre 0.8 g ▎ cholesterol 30 mg ▎ sodium 101 mg ▎ energy 198 kJ (47 Cal) ▎ GI low ▼

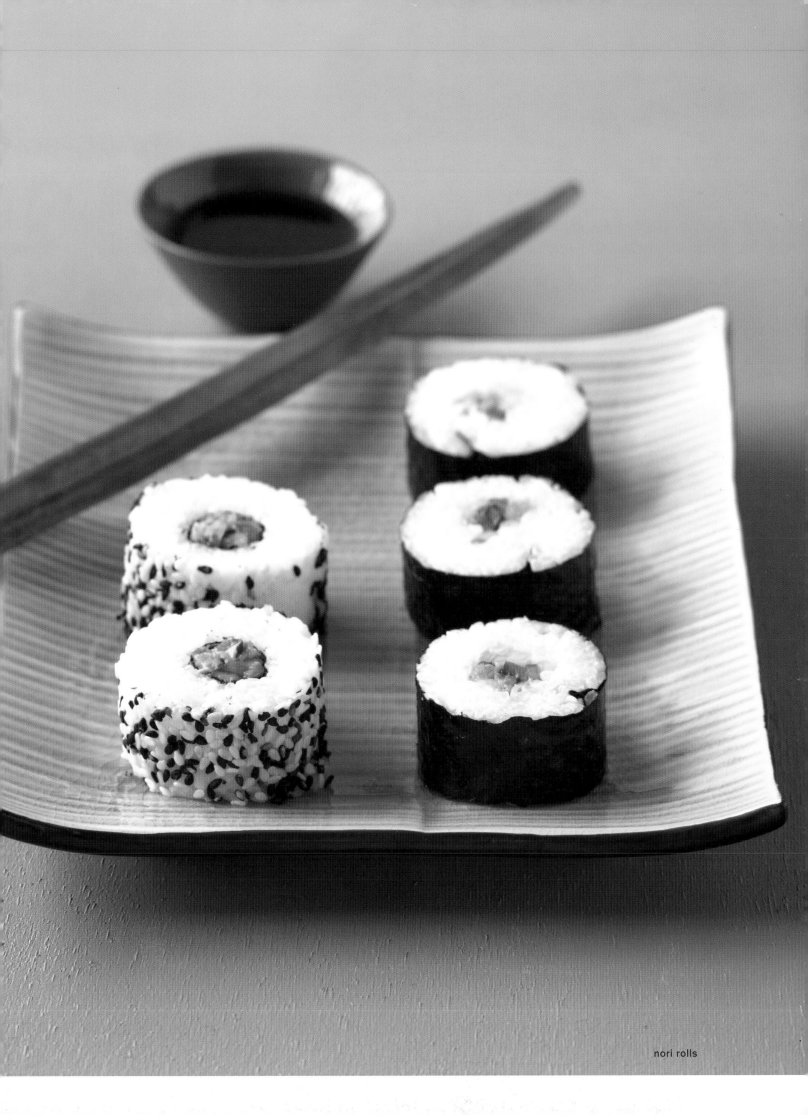

nori rolls

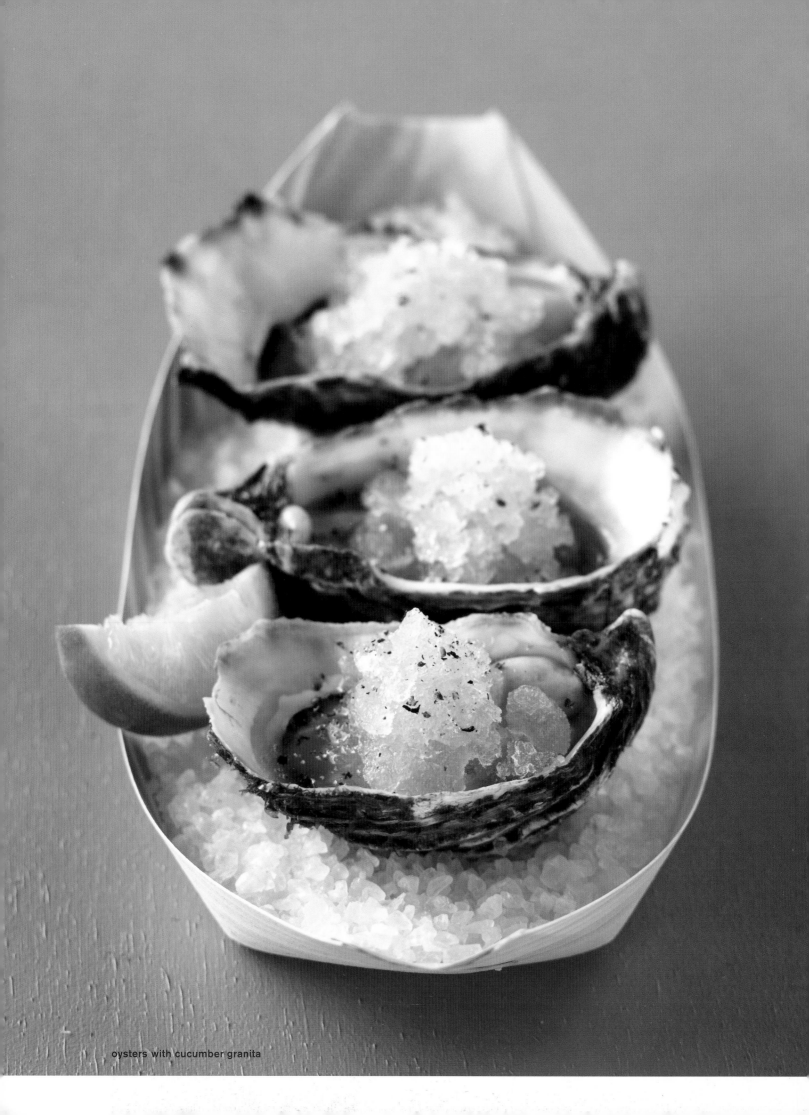

oysters with cucumber granita

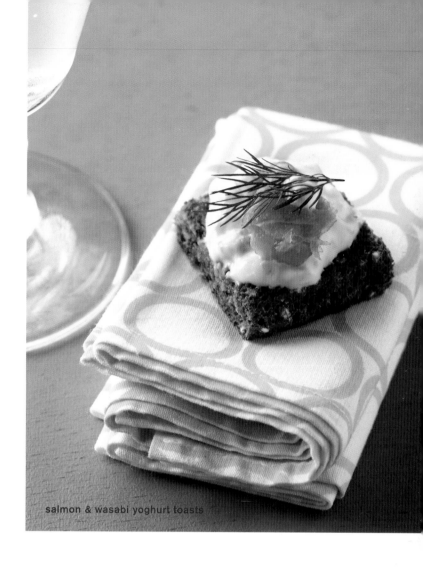

salmon & wasabi yoghurt toasts

oysters with cucumber granita makes 18

1 telegraph cucumber

1 celery stick

1 cup (250 ml/8 fl oz) sparkling mineral water

few splashes of Tabasco sauce

18 freshly shucked oysters on the shell

cracked black pepper

1 Push the cucumber and celery through a juice extractor. Pour into a jug, add the mineral water and Tabasco and mix to combine.

2 Pour the mixture into a shallow metal container and freeze until it starts to harden around the edges. Break up the crystals with a fork and return to the freezer for 1 hour. Repeat the whole process and freeze again.

3 Arrange the oysters on a platter and top with the granita and a little cracked black pepper. Serve with lime wedges.

per oyster fat 1.2 g ▌ saturated fat 0.4 g ▌ protein 6.3 g ▌ carbohydrate 0.6 g ▌ fibre 0.2 g ▌ cholesterol 40 mg ▌ sodium 165 mg ▌ energy 165 kJ (39 Cal) ▌ GI low ▽

salmon & wasabi yoghurt toasts makes 16

4 slices low-GI rye bread, toasted

1/2 cup (130 g/4 1/2 oz) low-fat Greek-style plain yoghurt

1/2 Lebanese cucumber, peeled and finely diced

1 teaspoon wasabi

50 g (1 2/3 oz) smoked salmon, cut into 3 cm (1 1/4 in) pieces

1 teaspoon fresh dill

1 Remove the crusts from the toasted bread and cut into quarters.

2 Put the yoghurt, cucumber and wasabi into a small bowl and mix well. Reserve 1 tablespoon.

3 Spread the wasabi yoghurt on the toasts. Top with a piece of folded salmon, a small dollop of the reserved yoghurt and a sprig of dill.

per toast fat 0.4 g ▌ saturated fat 0.1 g ▌ protein 2 g ▌ carbohydrate 4.6 g ▌ fibre 0.6 g ▌ cholesterol 2 mg ▌ sodium 116 mg ▌ energy 136 kJ (32 Cal) ▌ GI low ▽

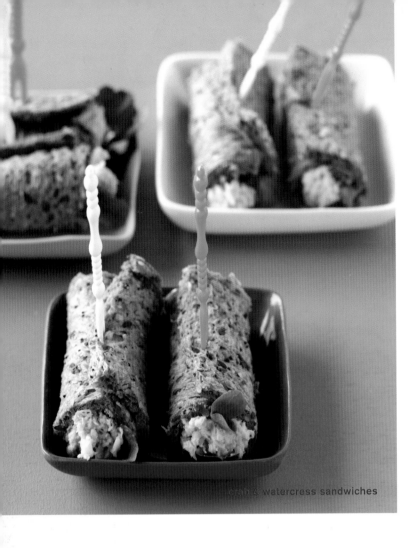
crab & watercress sandwiches

smoked chicken & enoki wraps makes 20

100 g (3¹/₃ oz) mung bean (glass) noodles	20 rice paper rounds, 18 cm (7 in) diameter
¹/₃ cup (80 ml/2²/₃ fl oz) hoisin sauce	4 spring onions (scallions), cut into short lengths
¹/₄ teaspoon five-spice powder	200 g (6¹/₂ oz) enoki mushrooms
¹/₄ teaspoon ground white pepper	1 Lebanese cucumber, unpeeled, cut into thin strips
300 g (10 oz) smoked boneless chicken breast, skin removed, sliced	

1 Put the noodles into a bowl, cover with boiling water and set aside for 10 minutes or until soft. Drain well.

2 Put the hoisin sauce, five-spice powder and pepper into a bowl and mix to combine. Add the chicken and mix well to coat in the sauce.

3 Soak a rice paper round in lukewarm water until soft, then place on a clean, dry tea towel. Top with some of the noodles, chicken, spring onions, mushrooms and cucumber. Roll up to enclose the filling, leaving some of the filling showing at the top. Cover with damp absorbent paper while you prepare the remaining wraps.

per wrap fat 1.4 g ▎ saturated fat 0.3 g ▎ protein 4.7 g ▎ carbohydrate 14.1 g ▎ fibre 0.9 g ▎ cholesterol 12 mg ▎ sodium 214 mg ▎ energy 379 kJ (91 Cal) ▎ GI low ▼

crab & watercress sandwiches makes 12

12 slices wholegrain bread	2 tablespoons low-fat mayonnaise
500 g (1 lb) fresh crab meat	1 teaspoon mustard powder
1 tablespoon low-fat Greek-style plain yoghurt	1 cup (30 g/1 oz) watercress sprigs

1 Remove the crusts from the bread and roll each slice with a rolling pin until very thin.

2 Put the crab meat, yoghurt, mayonnaise and mustard powder into a bowl and mix to combine.

3 Spoon a little of the crab filling along one edge of each slice of bread and top with a couple of sprigs of watercress. Roll up to enclose the filling and secure with toothpicks. Cover with a damp towel until ready to serve.

per sandwich fat 2 g ▎ saturated fat 0.4 g ▎ protein 10.3 g ▎ carbohydrate 10.9 g ▎ fibre 4.5 g ▎ cholesterol 35 mg ▎ sodium 281 mg ▎ energy 469 kJ (112 Cal) ▎ GI low ▼

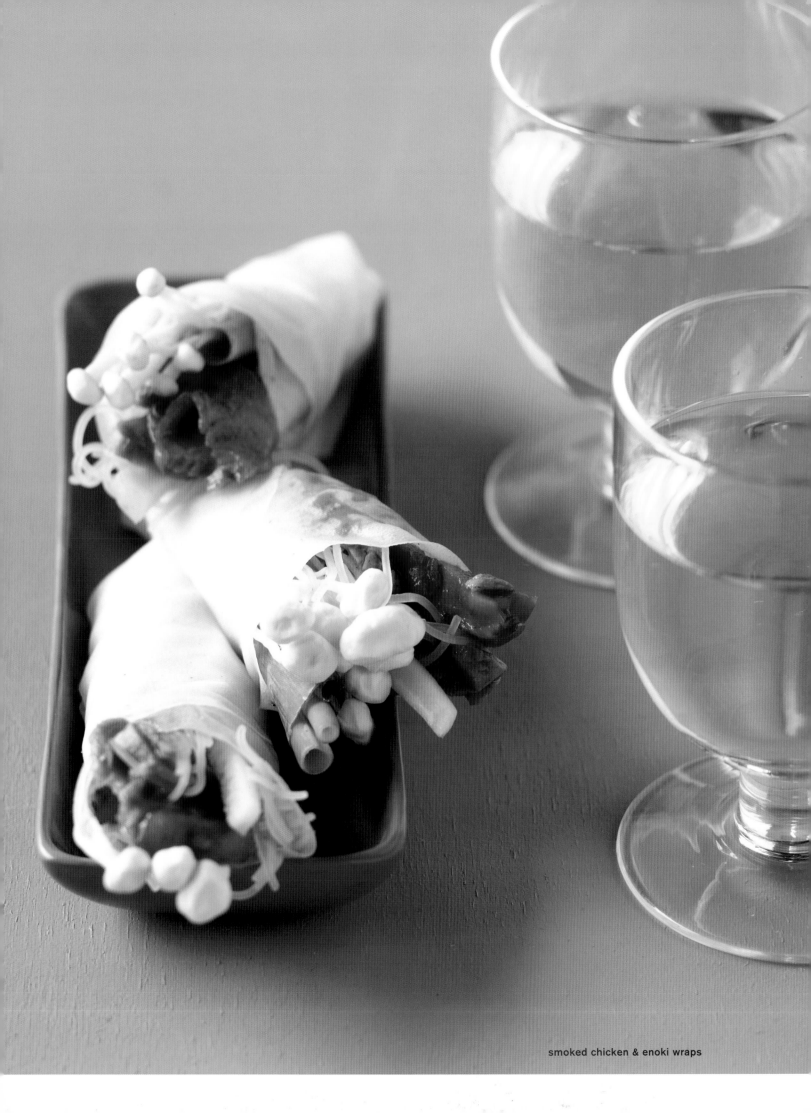

smoked chicken & enoki wraps

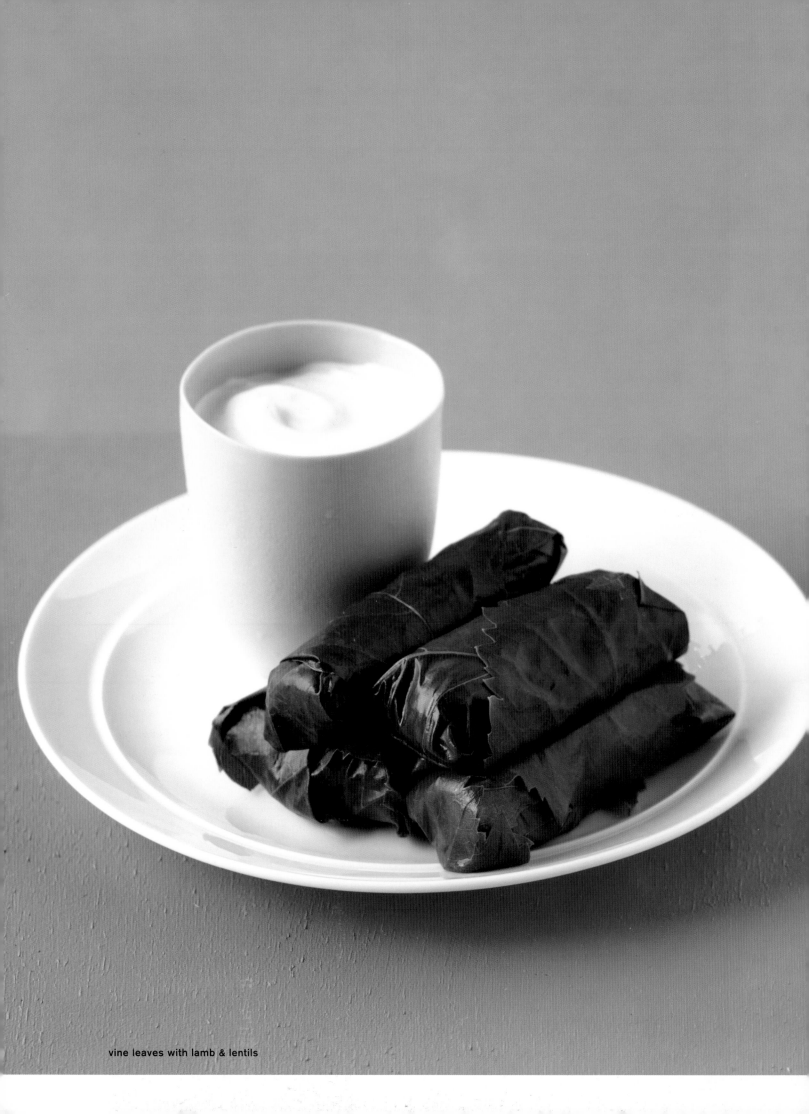

vine leaves with lamb & lentils

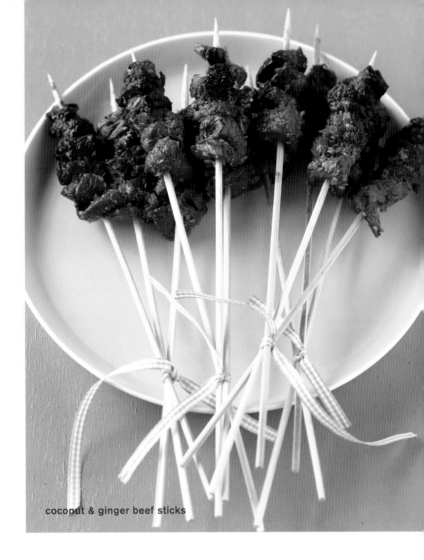

coconut & ginger beef sticks

vine leaves with lamb & lentils   makes 18

1 teaspoon olive oil
1/2 onion, finely chopped
50 g (1²/³ oz) lean lamb mince
1/4 cup (50 g/1²/³ oz) basmati rice
1/4 cup (45 g/1¹/² oz) canned brown lentils
1 cup (250 ml/8 fl oz) water
100 ml (3¹/³ fl oz) lemon juice
1/2 teaspoon ground black pepper
1 tablespoon fresh dill, chopped
1 tablespoon fresh mint, chopped
24 vine leaves in brine

1   Heat the oil in a fry pan over medium heat. Add the onion and lamb and cook for 10 minutes or until the onion is soft. Add the rice, lentils, water, 1/4 cup (60 ml/2 fl oz) of the lemon juice, pepper, dill and mint and bring to the boil. Reduce the heat to low and gently simmer for 10 minutes or until the water has evaporated. Set aside to cool.

2   Gently rinse the vine leaves and pat dry, reserving 6 leaves. Lay on a flat surface, stalk-side up. Place 1 tablespoon of the lentil mixture in the centre of each vine leaf, fold the top of the leaf over the mixture, then fold in the sides and roll up tightly.

3   Line a large saucepan with the reserved vine leaves and pack the rolls in a single layer. Pour over the remaining lemon juice and enough water to cover the rolls. Place a plate on top of the rolls to prevent them from opening. Cover and bring to the boil over high heat. Reduce the heat to low and simmer for 45 minutes or until heated through.

4   Drain the vine leaves. Serve cold with low-fat Greek-style plain yoghurt.

per roll fat 0.5 g ▮ saturated fat 0.1 g ▮ protein 1.1 g ▮ carbohydrate 2.8 g ▮ fibre 0.3 g ▮ cholesterol 2 mg ▮ sodium 82 mg ▮ energy 89 kJ (21 Cal) ▮ GI low ▼

coconut & ginger beef sticks   makes 16

500 g (1 lb) lean beef rump steak, cut into long thin strips
2 tablespoons kecap manis
1 tablespoon fish sauce
1 tablespoon lime juice
1/2 teaspoon sesame oil
2 cloves garlic, crushed
2 tablespoons grated fresh ginger
1 tablespoon desiccated coconut

1   Put the beef into a shallow non-metallic bowl. Add the kecap manis, fish sauce, lime juice, sesame oil, garlic, ginger and coconut and mix to combine. Cover and refrigerate for 4 hours or overnight.

2   Soak 16 bamboo skewers in water for 30 minutes.

3   Thread the beef onto the skewers. Cook on a lightly oiled chargrill for 3–5 minutes or until tender, turning several times during cooking.

per beef stick fat 1.8 g ▮ saturated fat 0.9 g ▮ protein 7 g ▮ carbohydrate 1 g ▮ fibre 0.1 g ▮ cholesterol 20 mg ▮ sodium 180 mg ▮ energy 205 kJ (49 Cal) ▮ GI low ▼

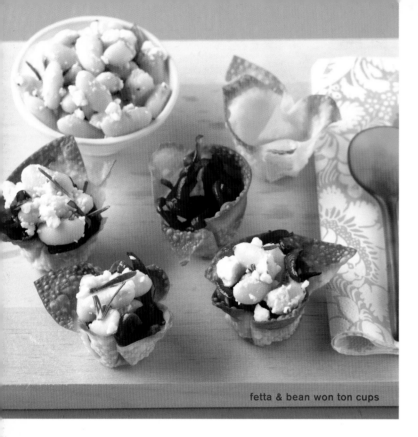

fetta & bean won ton cups

lemon grass & lime fish cakes makes 30

¼ cup (60 ml/2 fl oz) rice wine vinegar	4 kaffir lime leaves, thinly sliced
2 tablespoons lime juice	1 teaspoon grated lime zest
3 teaspoons grated palm sugar or brown sugar	2 teaspoons ground white pepper
1 large red chilli, finely chopped	1 tablespoon fish sauce
1 large green chilli, finely chopped	2 tablespoons chopped fresh coriander (cilantro)
500 g (1 lb) red fish fillets	100 g (3⅓ oz) snake beans, thinly sliced
3 tablespoons chopped lemon grass	2 tablespoons peanut oil

1 Preheat oven to 180°C (350°F/Gas 4). Line a baking tray with baking paper.

2 Put the vinegar, 1 tablespoon of the lime juice, 2 teaspoons of the sugar and the chillies into a bowl and mix to combine. Set the dipping sauce aside to allow the flavours to develop.

3 Meanwhile, put the fish, lemon grass, lime leaves, lime zest, pepper, fish sauce, coriander, remaining lime juice and remaining sugar into a food processor and process until combined.

4 Transfer the fish mixture to a bowl and stir in the beans. Shape tablespoons of the mixture into balls and flatten slightly. Refrigerate on the prepared tray for 1 hour or until firm.

5 Heat the oil in a fry pan over medium heat and cook the fish cakes in batches for 3 minutes each side or until cooked through. Place in the oven to keep warm while you cook the remaining fish cakes.

6 Serve the fish cakes with the dipping sauce.

per fish cake fat 0.7 g ▌ saturated fat 0.1 g ▌ protein 3 g
▌ carbohydrate 0.6 g ▌ fibre 0.2 g ▌ cholesterol 3 mg
▌ sodium 72 mg ▌ energy 93 kJ (22 Cal) ▌ GI low ▼

fetta & bean won ton cups makes 24

24 won ton wrappers	400 g (13 oz) can cannellini beans, rinsed and drained
olive oil spray	
2 red (Spanish) onions, thinly sliced	1 tablespoon chopped fresh rosemary
2 tablespoons balsamic vinegar	60 g (2 oz) low-fat fetta cheese
1 teaspoon brown sugar	2 teaspoons olive oil
2 tablespoons water	cracked black pepper

1 Preheat oven to 200°C (400°F/Gas 6).

2 Line 24 mini muffin holes with the won ton wrappers. Lightly spray with olive oil spray and bake for 10–15 minutes or until crisp and golden.

3 Put the onions, vinegar, sugar and water into a pan and cook over medium heat for 15 minutes or until the onions have caramelised.

4 Combine the beans, rosemary, fetta and olive oil and season with cracked black pepper.

5 Spoon a little of the onion mixture into the won ton cups, followed by the bean mixture. Garnish with small sprigs of thyme.

per cup fat 1 g ▌ saturated fat 0.3 g ▌ protein 2.3 g
▌ carbohydrate 6.7 g ▌ fibre 1 g ▌ cholesterol 1 mg
▌ sodium 75 mg ▌ energy 198 kJ (47 Cal) ▌ GI low–med ▼–◆

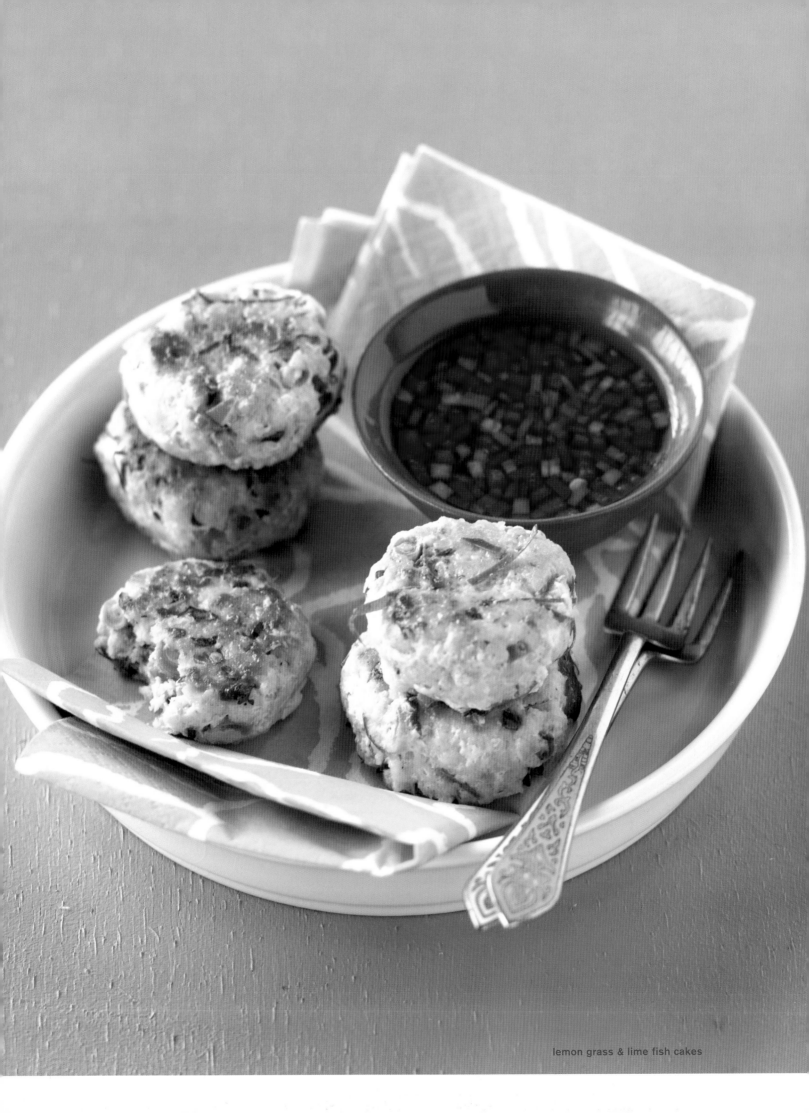

lemon grass & lime fish cakes

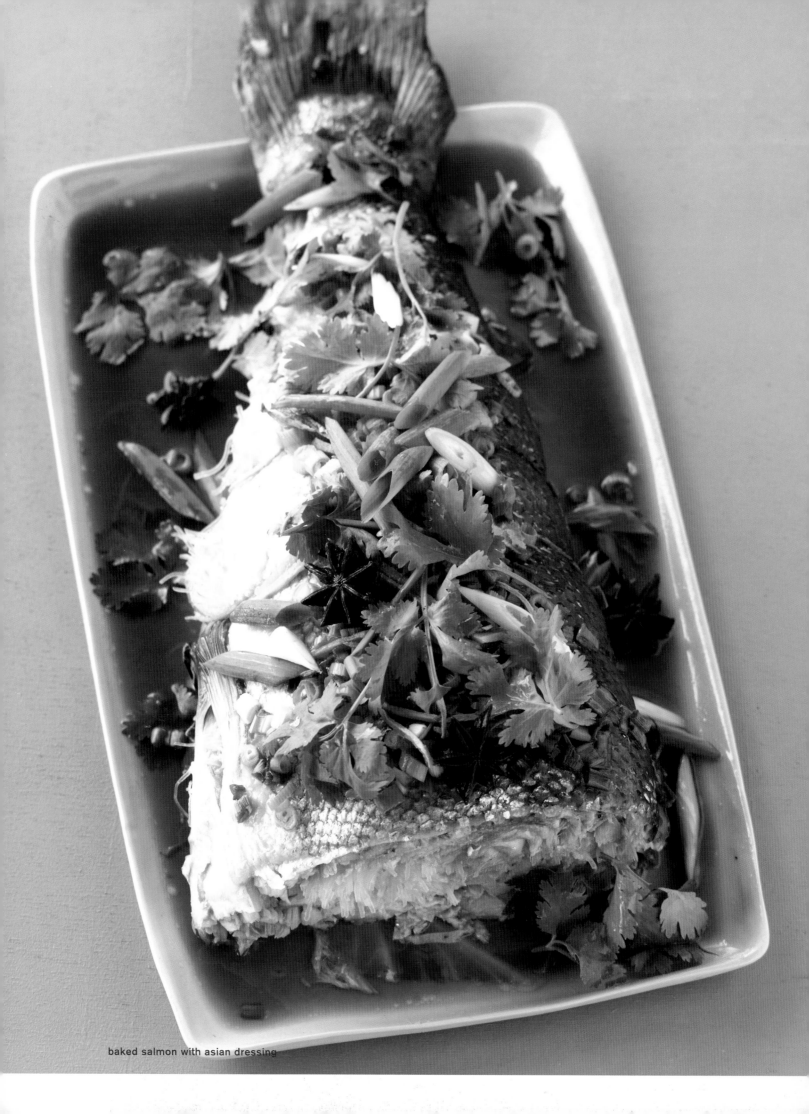

baked salmon with asian dressing

baked salmon with asian dressing serves 12

100 g (3¹/₃ oz) mung
   bean (glass) noodles
2 tablespoons chopped
   fresh coriander
   (cilantro)
2 tablespoons grated
   fresh ginger
2 teaspoons grated lime
   zest
2 tablespoons lime juice
¹/₂ teaspoon sesame oil
8 spring onions
   (scallions)
1 boned salmon (1 kg/
   2 lb)
6 large cabbage leaves

4 tablespoons finely
   shredded fresh ginger
1 cup (250 ml/8 fl oz)
   reduced-salt chicken
   stock
¹/₄ cup (60 ml/2 fl oz)
   Chinese rice wine
1 tablespoon reduced-
   salt soy sauce
1 tablespoon yellow box
   honey
2 star anise
1 cinnamon stick
1 cup (30 g/1 oz) fresh
   coriander (cilantro)

1 Preheat oven to 180°C (350°F/Gas 4).

2 Put the noodles into a bowl, cover with boiling water and set aside for 10 minutes or until soft. Drain and transfer to a bowl.

3 Add the chopped coriander, grated ginger, lime zest, lime juice and sesame oil to the noodles and mix to combine.

4 Thinly slice half the spring onions. Cut the rest of the spring onions into short lengths on the diagonal.

5 Fill the cavity of the salmon with the noodle mixture and secure with kitchen string. Arrange the salmon on the cabbage leaves on a wire rack in a roasting dish. Top with the shredded ginger and the thinly sliced spring onions, cover with lightly greased foil and bake for 40 minutes or until tender.

6 Meanwhile, put the chicken stock, rice wine, soy sauce, honey, star anise and cinnamon stick into a pan. Bring to the boil over high heat and cook for 10 minutes or until the liquid has reduced by half.

7 Serve the salmon on a large platter, drizzled with the sauce and sprinkled with the remaining spring onions and the coriander.

per serve fat 6.2 g ▮ saturated fat 1.4 g ▮ protein 17.3 g
▮ carbohydrate 11.1 g ▮ fibre 1 g ▮ cholesterol 44 mg
▮ sodium 157 mg ▮ energy 737 kJ (176 Cal) ▮ GI low ▼

▮ Replace the rice wine with extra stock, if preferred.

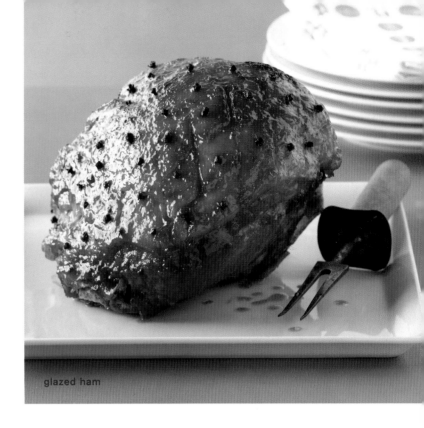
glazed ham

glazed ham serves 14–16

¹/₂ leg of ham (4 kg/8 lb)
4 cups (1 litre/32 fl oz)
   unsweetened low-GI
   apple juice
1 onion, halved
1 bay leaf

40 cloves
3 tablespoons no-added
   sugar apricot pure fruit
   spread
1 tablespoon mustard
   powder

1 Remove the rind and trim any excess fat from the ham, leaving a thin layer of fat on top. Score the fat in a diamond pattern, being careful not to cut all the way through the fat to the ham.

2 Put the ham into a large pan and add the apple juice, onion and bay leaf. Bring to the boil, then reduce the heat, cover and simmer for 1 hour. Remove the ham from the pan and set aside to cool slightly. Press the cloves into the ham.

3 Preheat oven to 200°C (400°F/Gas 6).

4 Strain 300 ml (10 fl oz) of the cooking liquid into a pan. Add the fruit spread and mustard powder. Bring to the boil and cook for 10 minutes or until thick and syrupy.

5 Brush the glaze over the ham and bake for 20 minutes or until the glaze is golden and bubbling. Trim the ham of fat before serving.

per serve (16) fat 9 g ▮ saturated fat 3.3 g ▮ protein 28.8 g
▮ carbohydrate 8.7 g ▮ fibre 0.3 g ▮ cholesterol 81 mg
▮ sodium 2423 mg ▮ energy 967 kJ (231 Cal) ▮ GI low ▼

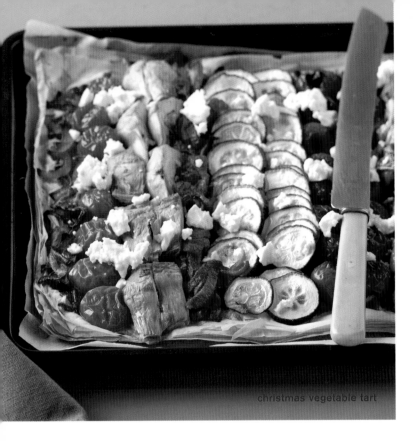
christmas vegetable tart

turkey breast with fruit stuffing serves 8–10

¹/₂ cup (70 g/2¹/₄ oz) bulgur wheat

pinch of saffron threads

1¹/₂ cups (375 ml/ 12 fl oz) boiling reduced-salt chicken stock

2 teaspoons olive oil

2 onions, sliced

1 teaspoon ground cumin

1 teaspoon ground cinnamon

1¹/₂ cups (100 g/3¹/₃ oz) fresh wholegrain breadcrumbs

¹/₂ cup (70 g/2¹/₄ oz) dried apricots, finely chopped

¹/₂ cup (90 g/3 oz) pitted prunes, finely chopped

2 teaspoons grated lemon zest

1 tablespoon chopped fresh sage

2 tablespoons chopped fresh parsley

3.5 kg (7 lb) turkey breast (ask your butcher to remove the bone); 2 kg (4 lb) with bone removed

1 Preheat oven to 180°C (350°F/Gas 4).

2 Put the bulgur wheat and saffron into a bowl. Add 1 cup (250 ml/8 fl oz) of the boiling chicken stock and set aside for 10 minutes or until all the liquid has been absorbed.

3 Heat the oil in a fry pan over medium heat. Add the onions and cook for 5 minutes or until soft. Add the cumin, cinnamon and the remaining stock and cook for 5 minutes.

4 Add the spiced onions, breadcrumbs, apricots, prunes, lemon zest, sage and parsley to the bulgur wheat and mix well to combine.

5 Place the turkey, skin-side down, on a board. Spoon the stuffing along the centre. Fold the breast in and tie up using kitchen string.

6 Place the turkey on a rack over simmering water in a baking dish. Bake for 1–1¹/₂ hours or until the turkey is cooked through. Set aside for 10 minutes before removing the skin and slicing. Serve with gravy (page 120).

per serve (10) fat 6.5 g ▮ saturated fat 1.3 g ▮ protein 40.3 g ▮ carbohydrate 17 g ▮ fibre 3.6 g ▮ cholesterol 83 mg ▮ sodium 417 mg ▮ energy 1243 kJ (297 Cal) ▮ GI low ▼

christmas vegetable tart serves 12

2 teaspoons olive oil

4 onions, sliced

8 sheets filo pastry

olive oil spray

250 g (8 oz) cherry tomatoes

2 zucchini (courgette), thinly sliced

100 g (3¹/₃ oz) roast capsicum (bell pepper), sliced

200 g (6¹/₂ oz) marinated artichokes

100 g (3¹/₃ oz) low-fat fetta cheese, crumbled

1 Preheat oven to 200°C (400°F/Gas 6). Line a large baking tray with baking paper.

2 Heat the oil in a fry pan over medium heat. Add the onions and cook for 10 minutes or until caramelised. Set aside to cool.

3 Place one sheet of filo pastry on the prepared tray, lightly spray with olive oil and top with another sheet of pastry. Repeat with the remaining pastry.

4 Spread the onions over the pastry, leaving a 2 cm (³/4 in) border. Arrange the tomatoes, zucchini, capsicum and artichokes in rows on the pastry.

5 Bake the tart for 30 minutes or until the pastry is crisp and golden. Sprinkle with the fetta and serve.

per serve fat 2.7 g ▮ saturated fat 1 g ▮ protein 4 g ▮ carbohydrate 8.1 g ▮ fibre 1.8 g ▮ cholesterol 2 mg ▮ sodium 213 mg ▮ energy 322 kJ (77 Cal) ▮ GI low–med ▼–◆

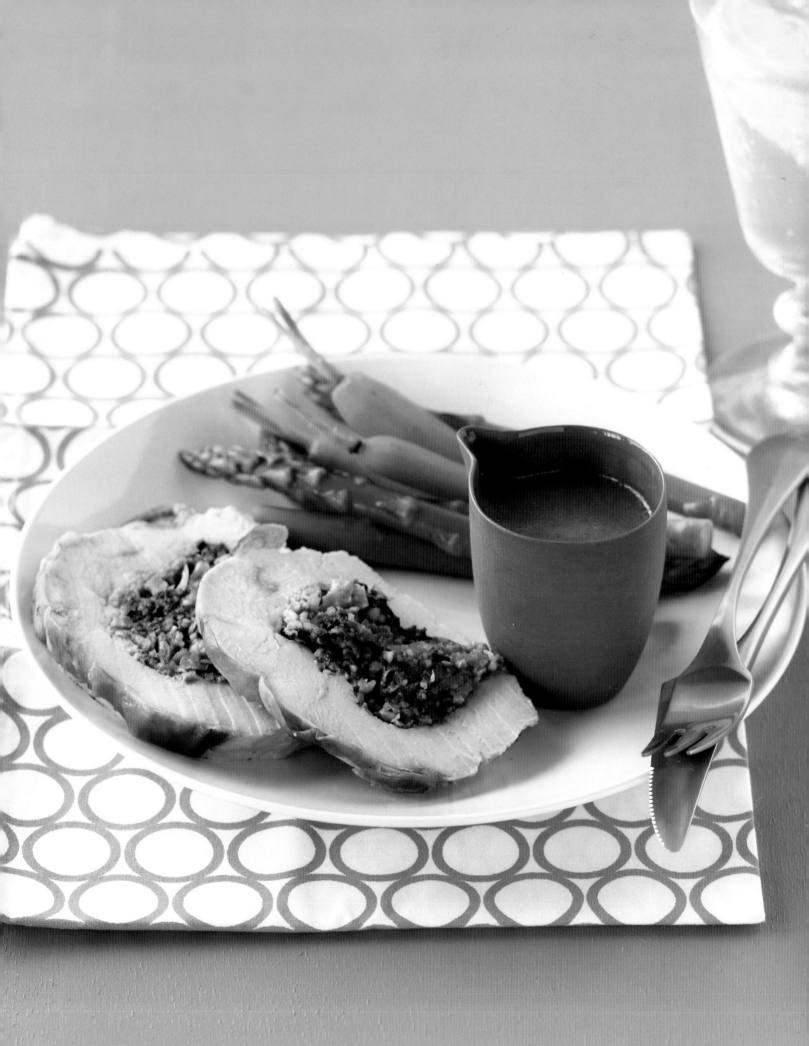

turkey breast with fruit stuffing

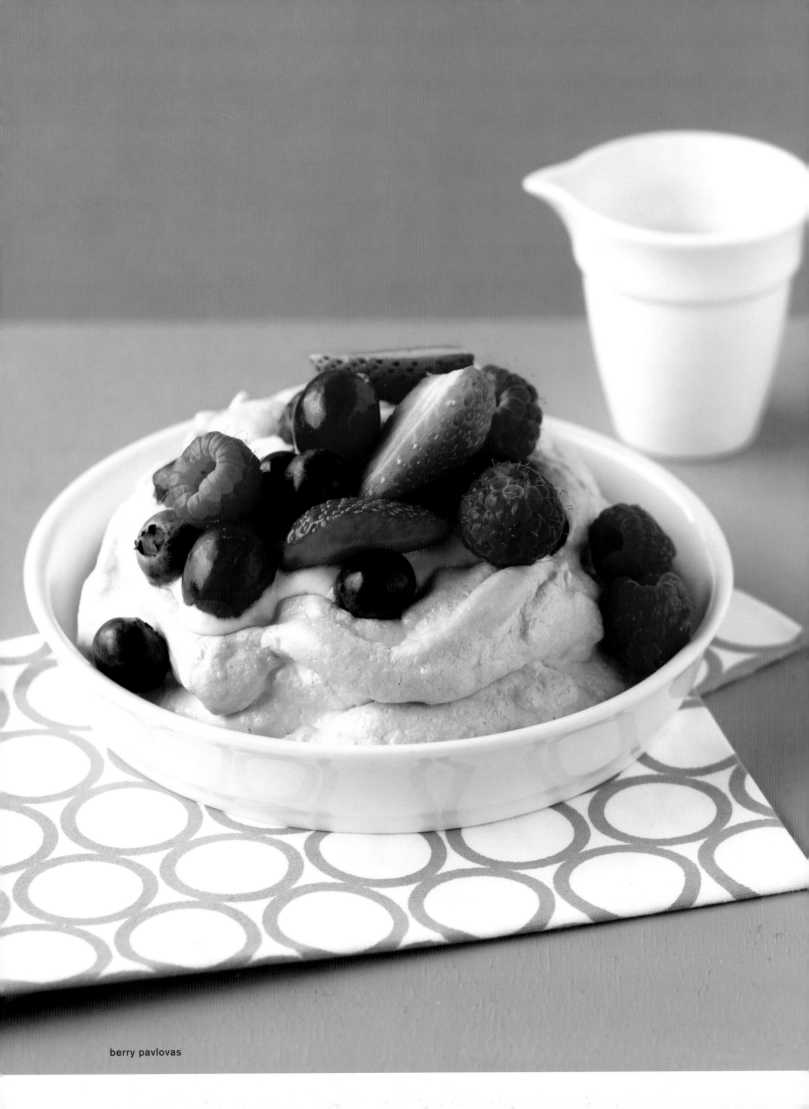

berry pavlovas

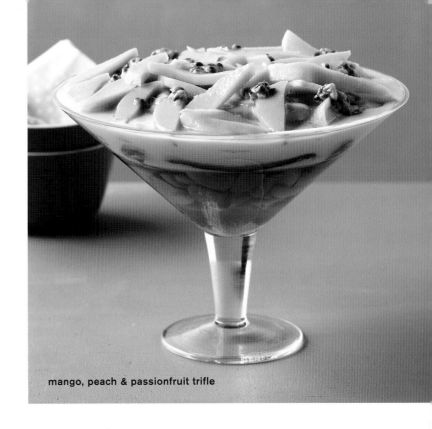

mango, peach & passionfruit trifle

berry pavlovas serves 8

6 egg whites, lightly
 beaten
1½ cups (38 g/1¼ oz)
 low-calorie sweetener
 suitable for baking
300 g (10 oz) low-fat
 Greek-style plain
 yoghurt

1 cup (250 ml/8 fl oz)
 low-fat vanilla custard
1 teaspoon rosewater
200 g (6½ oz) fresh
 mixed berries
200 g (6½ oz) seedless
 black grapes

1 Preheat oven to 180°C (350°F/Gas 4). Line a baking tray with baking paper.
2 Whisk the egg whites in a clean, dry bowl until soft peaks form. Gradually add the sweetener and beat until stiff peaks form.
3 Drop spoonfuls of the meringue onto the prepared tray and shape into 8 circles. Smooth the sides using a flat-bladed knife. Bake for 15 minutes, then reduce the oven to 120°C (250°F/Gas ½) and bake for 1½ hours or until the pavlovas are crisp and dry. Cool in the oven with the door ajar.
4 Put the yoghurt, custard and rosewater into a bowl and gently mix to combine.
5 Serve the pavlovas topped with the yoghurt mixture, berries and grapes.

per serve fat 0.4 g ▌ saturated fat 0.2 g ▌ protein 6.7 g ▌ carbohydrate 15.7 g ▌ fibre 0.8 g ▌ cholesterol 4 mg ▌ sodium 87 mg ▌ energy 405 kJ (97 Cal) ▌ GI low ▼

mango, peach & passionfruit trifle serves 12

1 packet (10 g/⅓ oz)
 low-joule pineapple
 jelly
400 g (13 oz) can
 peaches in natural
 juice, drained and
 roughly chopped
10 passionfruit

2 cups (500 ml/16 fl oz)
 low-GI apple,
 passionfruit and
 pineapple juice
200 g (6½ oz) thick
 sponge finger biscuits
2 cups (500 ml/16 fl oz)
 low-fat vanilla custard
2 mangoes, sliced

1 Prepare the jelly following the manufacturer's instructions. Stir in the peaches. Pour into a serving dish and chill for 2 hours or until firmly set.
2 Heat the passionfruit and the juice in a pan until just warm. Transfer to a bowl.
3 Dip the biscuits into the juice mixture and arrange over the jelly. Reserve the remaining juice mixture.
4 Pour the custard over the biscuits. Top with the mangoes and the reserved juice mixture. Cover and refrigerate overnight.

per serve fat 1.3 g ▌ saturated fat 0.5 g ▌ protein 4.8 g ▌ carbohydrate 29.2 g ▌ fibre 3.1 g ▌ cholesterol 28 mg ▌ sodium 72 mg ▌ energy 644 kJ (154 Cal) ▌ GI low–med ▼–◆

▌ Enjoy in moderation as an occasional treat. Replace the juice with unsweetened apple juice, if preferred.

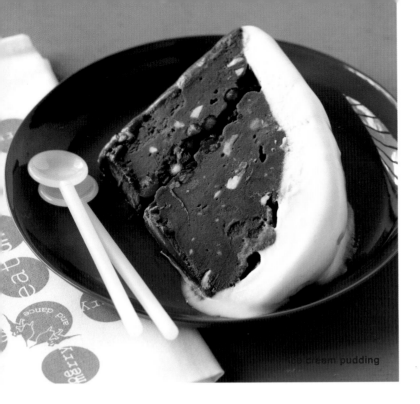

ice cream pudding

ice cream pudding serves 12

8 cups (2 litres/64 fl oz) low-GI low-fat vanilla ice cream

8 cups (2 litres/64 fl oz) low-GI low-fat chocolate ice cream

3 tablespoons chopped toasted hazelnuts

200 g (6½ oz) frozen mixed berries

1 Line a 16 cup (4 litre/128 fl oz) capacity pudding basin with plastic wrap, allowing it to overhang the side. Chill the basin in the freezer for 4 hours.

2 Slightly soften the vanilla ice cream and smooth it over the inside of the basin. Freeze until the ice cream is firm. Check the ice cream occasionally to make sure it has not run down the side.

3 Soften the chocolate ice cream and put it into a bowl. Add the hazelnuts and mix to combine. Spoon half the mixture into the basin and top with the berries and the remaining ice cream. Smooth the top, cover with plastic wrap and freeze overnight.

4 Invert the pudding onto a chilled plate and freeze until 5 minutes before serving. Cut the pudding into slices using a warm knife.

per serve fat 7.2 g ▌ saturated fat 3.7 g ▌ protein 8 g ▌ carbohydrate 44.7 g ▌ fibre 0.7 g ▌ cholesterol 16 mg ▌ sodium 161 mg ▌ energy 1153 kJ (275 Cal) ▌ GI low ▼

▌Enjoy in moderation as an occasional treat.

quick-mix christmas cake serves 16

2 cups (350 g/12 oz) dried mixed fruit

2 cups (340 g/11¼ oz) sultanas

1 cup (135 g/4¼ oz) dried apricots, roughly chopped

120 g (4 oz) reduced-fat margarine

½ cup (80 g/2⅔ oz) brown sugar or ½ cup (13 g/½ oz) low-calorie sweetener suitable for baking

1½ cups (375 ml/ 12 fl oz) unsweetened low-GI apple juice

1 cup (160 g/5⅓ oz) stone-ground plain flour

1 cup (160 g/5⅓ oz) stone-ground self-raising flour

2 teaspoons mixed spice

½ cup (55 g/1⅔ oz) almond meal

2 eggs, lightly beaten

1 Preheat oven to 160°C (315°F/Gas 2–3). Grease a 20 cm (8 in) deep round cake tin and line with 2 layers of baking paper.

2 Put the fruit, margarine, sugar or sweetener and apple juice into a pan. Simmer over low heat for 5 minutes or until the sugar has dissolved and the margarine has melted. Remove from the heat and set aside to cool.

3 Sift the flours and mixed spice into a bowl, stir in the almond meal and make a well in the centre.

4 Add the fruit and eggs to the dry ingredients and mix to combine. Spoon the mixture into the prepared tin and smooth the top with wet fingers. Wrap the tin in several layers of newspaper and secure them with kitchen string.

5 Bake the cake for 1½ hours or until it starts to come away from the side of the tin. Cool completely in the tin.

per serve (sugar) fat 6 g ▌ saturated fat 0.9 g ▌ protein 5 g ▌ carbohydrate 55.9 g ▌ fibre 4 g ▌ cholesterol 23 mg ▌ sodium 110 mg ▌ energy 1257 kJ (300 Cal) ▌ GI low ▼

per serve (sweetener) fat 6 g ▌ saturated fat 0.9 g ▌ protein 4.9 g ▌ carbohydrate 51.7 g ▌ fibre 4 g ▌ cholesterol 23 mg ▌ sodium 109 mg ▌ energy 1190 kJ (284 Cal) ▌ GI low ▼

▌Enjoy in moderation as an occasional treat.

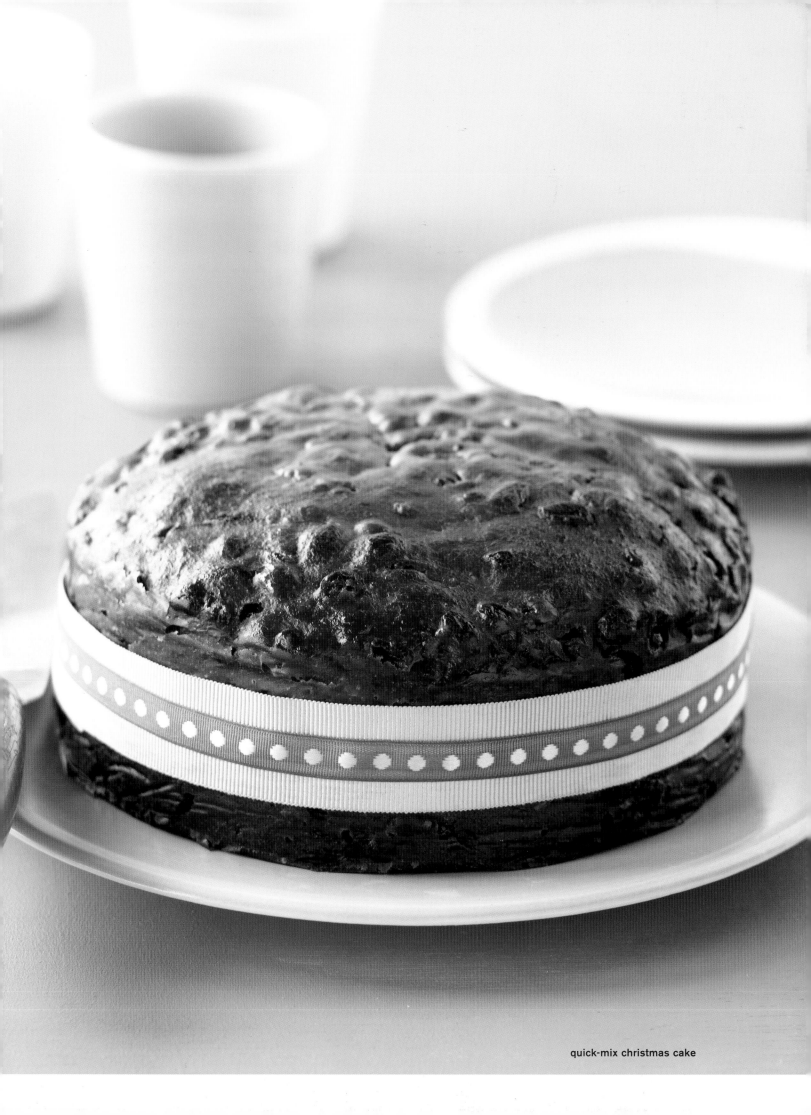

quick-mix christmas cake

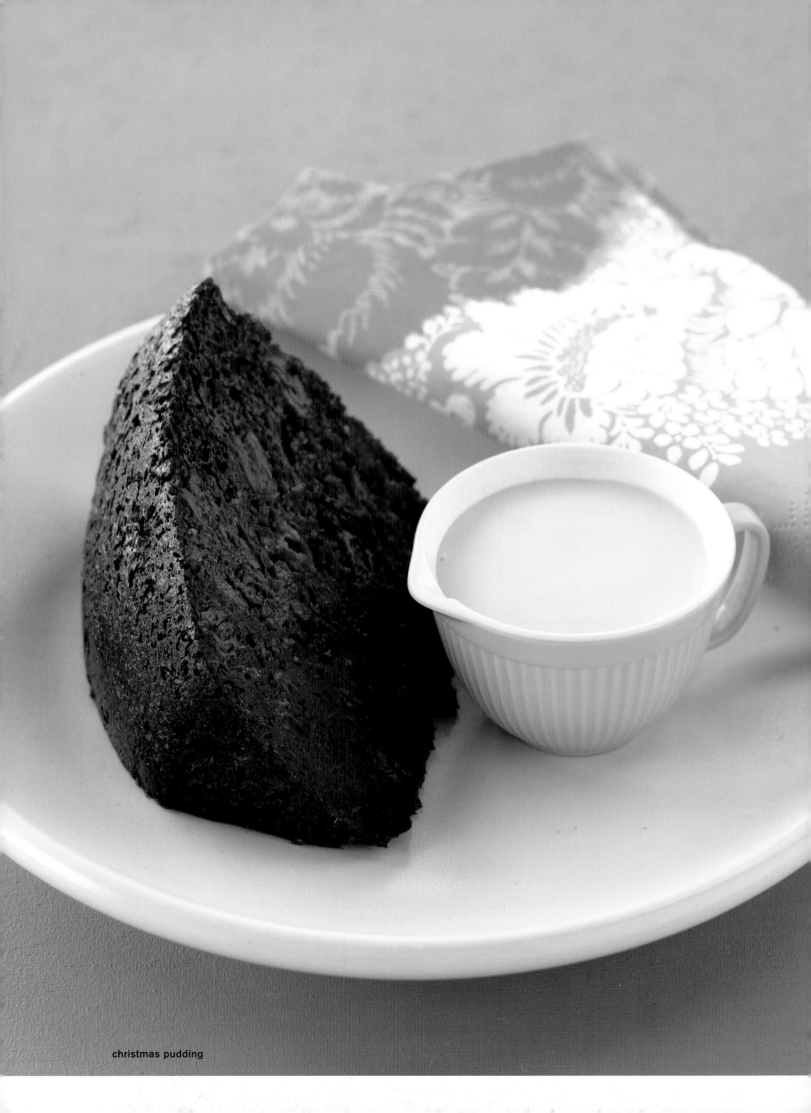

christmas pudding

christmas pudding serves 12

1 cup (135 g/4^1/$_2$ oz) dried fruit medley

1 cup (180 g/6 oz) pitted prunes, chopped

150 ml (5 fl oz) unsweetened low-GI apple juice

90 g (3 oz) stone-ground self-raising flour

1^1/$_2$ teaspoons bicarbonate of soda

2 teaspoons mixed spice

1 teaspoon ground ginger

3 eggs, lightly beaten

^{1}/$_2$ cup (80 g/2^2/$_3$ oz) brown sugar or

^{1}/$_2$ cup (13 g/^{1}/$_2$ oz) low-calorie sweetener suitable for baking

30 g (1 oz) reduced-fat olive oil margarine, melted

2 teaspoons grated orange zest

1 cup (65 g/2 oz) fresh wholegrain breadcrumbs

1 apple, peeled and grated

1 Lightly grease an 8 cup (2 litre/64 fl oz) pudding basin. Line the base with a circle of baking paper. Lay a sheet of baking paper on a sheet of foil and grease the paper. Make a fold down the centre.

2 Put the fruit medley and prunes into a bowl. Add the apple juice and set aside for 2 hours.

3 Sift the flour, bicarbonate of soda, mixed spice and ginger into a bowl. Add the fruit mixture and the remaining ingredients and mix well to combine.

4 Spoon the mixture into the prepared pudding basin. Cover with the paper and foil, paper-side down. Tie around the rim with kitchen string and then tie a handle on top of the basin. Put the basin onto a rack in a large pan. Pour in enough boiling water to come halfway up the side of the basin.

5 Cover the pan and bring to the boil. Reduce the heat and cook at a slow boil for 6 hours, adding more water when necessary.

6 To serve, reheat the pudding in a large saucepan of boiling water for 1^1/$_2$ hours, or reheat in the microwave. Serve with low-fat vanilla custard or low-GI low-fat vanilla ice cream.

per serve (sugar) fat 3.2 g ▌ saturated fat 1.1 g ▌ protein 3.6 g ▌ carbohydrate 30.7 g ▌ fibre 2.9 g ▌ cholesterol 47 mg ▌ sodium 269 mg ▌ energy 706 kJ (169 Cal) ▌ GI low ▽

per serve (sweetener) fat 3.2 g ▌ saturated fat 1.1 g ▌ protein 3.6 g ▌ carbohydrate 25.2 g ▌ fibre 2.9 g ▌ cholesterol 47 mg ▌ sodium 269 mg ▌ energy 619 kJ (148 Cal) ▌ GI low ▽

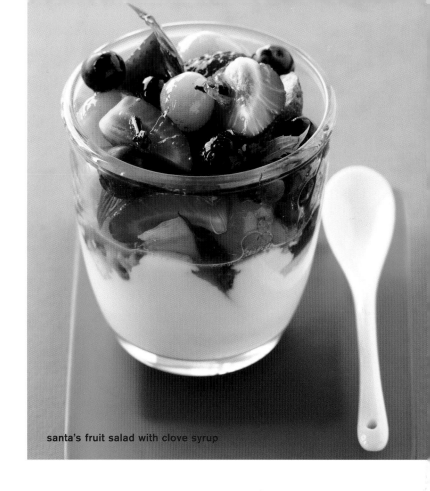

santa's fruit salad with clove syrup

santa's fruit salad with clove syrup serves 8

800 g (1 lb 10 oz) low-fat Greek-style plain yoghurt

3 peaches, sliced

3 nectarines, sliced

1 mango, cut into cubes

3 passionfruit

200 g (6^1/$_2$ oz) seedless green grapes

200 g (6^1/$_2$ oz) strawberries, chopped

150 g (5 oz) blueberries

^{1}/$_2$ cup (25 g/1 oz) fresh mint

^{1}/$_3$ cup (80 ml/2^2/$_3$ fl oz) pure maple syrup

^{1}/$_3$ cup (80 ml/2^2/$_3$ fl oz) unsweetened low-GI apple juice

8 cloves

2 teaspoons grated orange zest

1 Divide the yoghurt among 8 glasses. Put the peaches, nectarines, mango and passionfruit into a bowl and mix to combine. Spoon over the yoghurt and top with the combined grapes, berries and mint.

2 Put the maple syrup, apple juice, cloves and orange zest into a pan. Bring to the boil over high heat and cook for 5 minutes or until syrupy.

3 Drizzle the syrup over each fruit salad.

per serve fat 0.5 g ▌ saturated fat 0.1 g ▌ protein 8.3 g ▌ carbohydrate 34 g ▌ fibre 4.8 g ▌ cholesterol 5 mg ▌ sodium 79 mg ▌ energy 787 kJ (188 Cal) ▌ GI low ▽

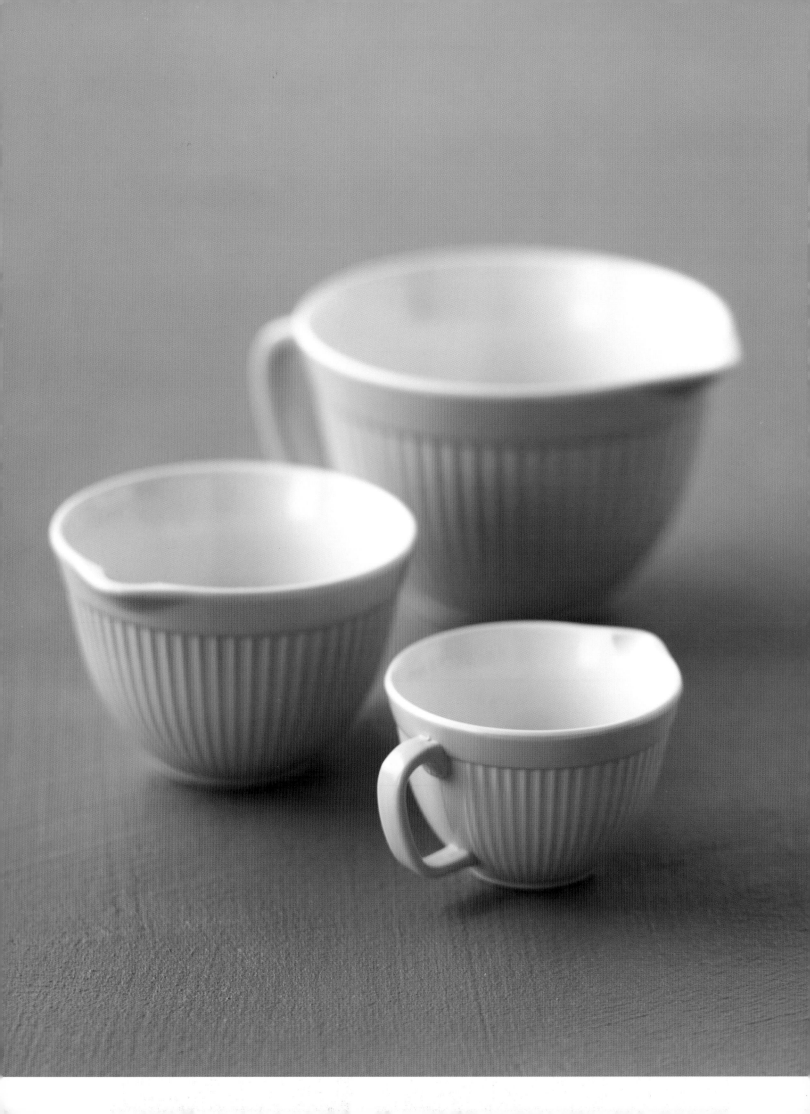

basics

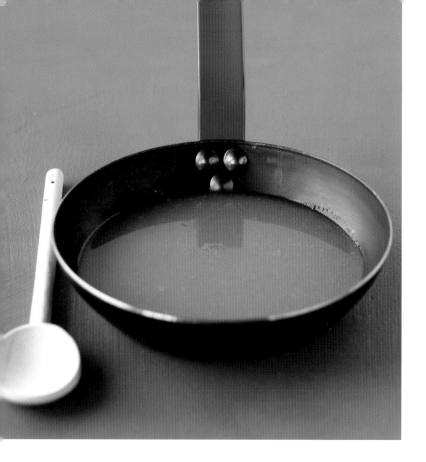
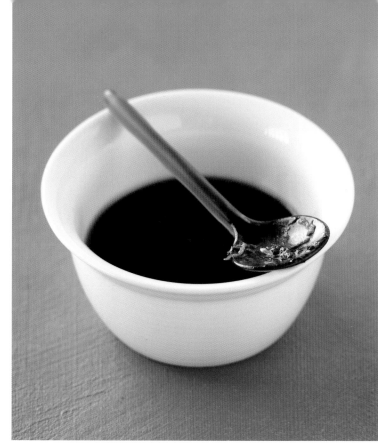

gravy makes 2 cups

2 tablespoons pan juices from roast or pan-fried meat or chicken

2 tablespoons stone-ground wholemeal plain flour

2 cups (500 ml/16 fl oz) reduced-salt chicken stock

1 Remove the meat or chicken from the roasting pan. Add the flour and stir to form a smooth paste. Cook, stirring, for 1 minute to remove any cooked sediment from the base of the roasting pan.

2 Remove the pan from the heat and gradually add the stock, stirring until smooth.

3 Return to the heat and cook, stirring constantly, until the gravy boils and thickens.

per tablespoon fat 0.03 g ▌ saturated fat 0.01 g ▌ protein 0.4 g ▌ carbohydrate 0.8 g ▌ fibre 0.03 g ▌ cholesterol 1 mg ▌ sodium 86 mg ▌ energy 21 kJ (5 Cal)

basic marinade makes ¹/₂ cup

¼ cup (60 ml/2 fl oz) reduced-salt soy sauce

1 tablespoon yellow box honey

1 tablespoon lemon or lime juice

1 teaspoon sesame oil

1 tablespoon grated fresh ginger

1 Put the soy sauce, honey, lemon or lime juice, sesame oil and ginger into a non-metallic bowl and mix to combine.

per tablespoon fat 0.8 g ▌ saturated fat 0.1 g ▌ protein 0.6 g ▌ carbohydrate 4.4 g ▌ fibre 0 g ▌ cholesterol 0 mg ▌ sodium 384 mg ▌ energy 115 kJ (27 Cal)

▌ Use the mixture to marinate 500 g (1 lb) of chicken, beef or pork in the refrigerator for at least 4 hours.

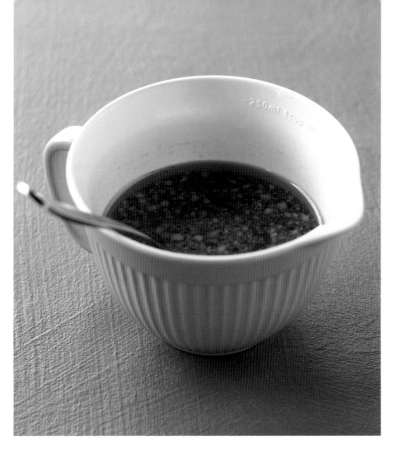
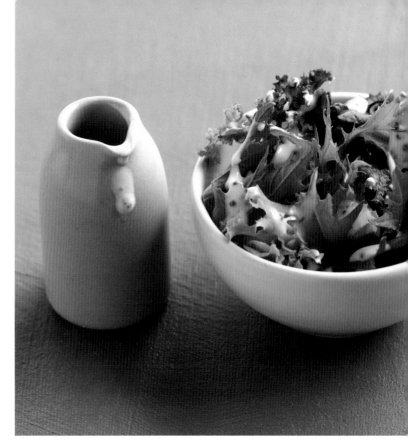

salad dressing makes ¹/₂ cup

2 cloves garlic, crushed
1 teaspoon wholegrain
    mustard
2 tablespoons lemon
    juice
2 teaspoons balsamic
    vinegar

1 teaspoon yellow box
    honey
¹/₄ cup (60 ml/2 fl oz)
    unsweetened low-GI
    apple juice
1 tablespoon extra virgin
    olive oil

1 Put the garlic, mustard, lemon juice, vinegar,
honey, apple juice and olive oil into a jug and whisk
to combine.

per tablespoon fat 2.4 g ▌saturated fat 0.3 g ▌protein 0.1 g

▌carbohydrate 1.8 g ▌fibre 0.1 g ▌cholesterol 0 mg

▌sodium 12 mg ▌energy 124 kJ (30 Cal)

▌Serve the dressing drizzled over a green salad.

creamy salad dressing makes ¹/₂ cup

¹/₃ cup (85 g/2³/₄ oz)
    low-fat Greek-style
    plain yoghurt
2 teaspoons wholegrain
    mustard

1 clove garlic, crushed
1 teaspoon yellow box
    honey
1 tablespoon rice wine
    vinegar

1 Put the yoghurt, mustard, garlic, honey and
vinegar into a bowl and whisk to combine.

per tablespoon fat 0.1 g ▌saturated fat 0 g ▌protein 1 g

▌carbohydrate 1.9 g ▌fibre 0.1 g ▌cholesterol 1 mg

▌sodium 24 mg ▌energy 56 kJ (13 Cal)

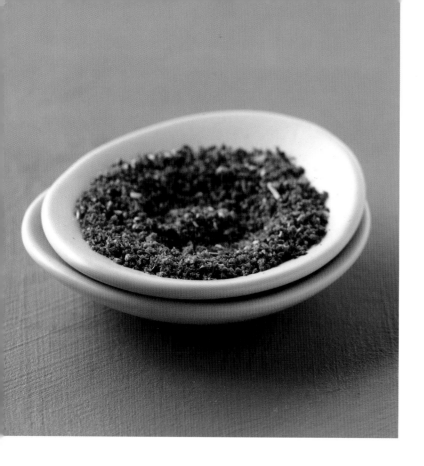
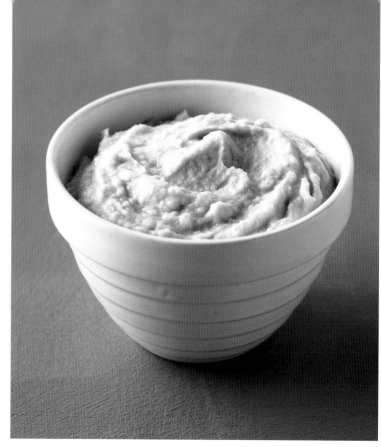

crumb coating makes 2 cups

6 slices dense
  wholegrain bread
1 teaspoon dried mixed
  herbs

2 tablespoons finely
  grated parmesan
  cheese
cracked black pepper

1 Toast the bread until crisp and golden. Cool completely, then break into small pieces. Place into a food processor and process until small crumbs form.
2 Add the dried herbs, parmesan and cracked black pepper and process until fine crumbs form.

per serve (4) fat 2.6 g ▌ saturated fat 0.9 g ▌ protein 6.1 g ▌ carbohydrate 21.9 g ▌ fibre 2.7 g ▌ cholesterol 3 mg ▌ sodium 309 mg ▌ energy 593 kJ (142 Cal)

▌ Use the crumb coating to coat 500 g (1 lb) of chicken, fish or veal that has been dusted with flour and dipped in egg white. Spray lightly with olive oil spray and bake at 180°C (350°F/Gas 4) until crisp and golden.

bean mash makes 2 cups

800 g (1 lb 10 oz) can
  cannellini beans,
  rinsed and drained
1 onion, halved
1 bay leaf

1 cup (250 ml/8 fl oz)
  reduced-salt chicken
  stock
cracked black pepper

1 Put the beans, onion, bay leaf and stock into a pan. Bring to the boil, then reduce the heat and simmer over medium heat for 10 minutes or until most of the liquid has been absorbed.
2 Discard the onion and bay leaf. Transfer the beans and any remaining liquid to a food processor and process until fairly smooth. Season with cracked black pepper.

per serve (4) fat 0.6 g ▌ saturated fat 0.2 g ▌ protein 11.7 g ▌ carbohydrate 19.8 g ▌ fibre 9.1 g ▌ cholesterol 1 mg ▌ sodium 162 mg ▌ energy 596 kJ (142 Cal)

▌ Serve the bean mash as a delicious lower-GI alternative to mashed potato.

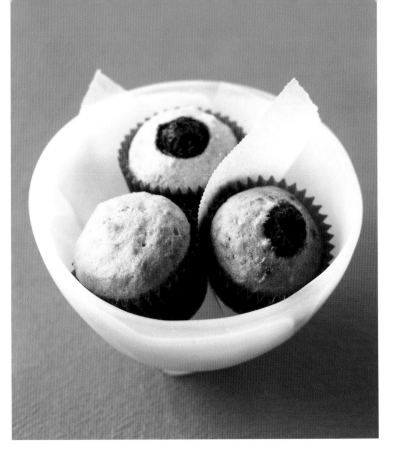

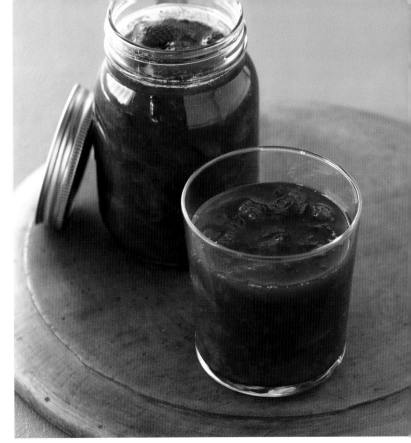

muffins makes 12

2 cups (320 g/10²/₃ oz)
  stone-ground
  wholemeal plain flour
2 teaspoons baking
  powder
¼ cup (35 g/1 oz)
  unprocessed oat bran
⅓ cup (50 g/1²/₃ oz)
  brown sugar

1 cup (160 g/5¹/₃ oz)
  semolina
3 eggs, lightly beaten
1½ cups (375 ml/
  12 fl oz) low-fat milk
2 tablespoons
  sunflower oil
140 g (4½ oz)
  unsweetened apple
  puree

1 Preheat oven to 180°C (350°F/Gas 4). Line 12 x
⅓ cup (80 ml/2²/₃ fl oz) capacity muffin holes.
2 Sift the flour and baking powder into a bowl. Stir
in the oat bran, sugar and semolina. Make a well in
the centre. Whisk together the eggs, milk, oil and
apple. Pour into the well and mix until just combined.
3 Divide the mixture among the muffin holes and
bake for 20–25 minutes or until risen and golden.

per muffin fat 5.3 g ▌ saturated fat 0.9 g ▌ protein 8 g
▌ carbohydrate 34.3 g ▌ fibre 4.1 g ▌ cholesterol 48 mg
▌ sodium 114 mg ▌ energy 942 kJ (225 Cal)

▌ To make berry muffins, push a berry into the top of
each muffin before baking.

strawberry jam makes 3 cups

750 g (1½ lb)
  strawberries, hulled
1 green apple, peeled
  and grated
2 tablespoons yellow
  box honey

1 vanilla bean, halved
  lengthwise
50 g (1²/₃ oz) jam setting
  mixture with pectin

1 Put the strawberries, apple, honey and vanilla
bean into a saucepan. Cook over medium heat for
15 minutes or until the strawberries are soft.
2 Add the jam setting mixture and bring to the
boil. Cook for 5 minutes, stirring often to prevent
the jam from sticking to the pan. Bottle the jam in
sterilised jars.

per tablespoon fat 0.03 g ▌ saturated fat 0 g ▌ protein 0.4 g
▌ carbohydrate 3.3 g ▌ fibre 0.6 g ▌ cholesterol 0 mg
▌ sodium 4 mg ▌ energy 66 kJ (16 Cal)

▌ This jam has a low sugar content so it needs to be
kept in the refrigerator. It will not keep for as long as
regular jams.

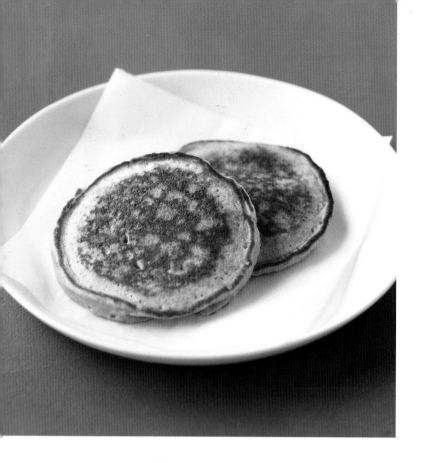

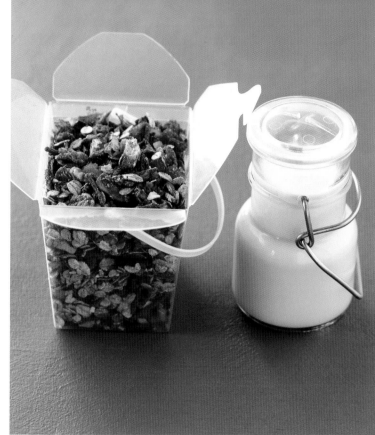

pancakes   makes 12

1 1/2 cups (240 g/7 2/3 oz)
    stone-ground
    wholemeal self-raising
    flour
1 teaspoon baking powder
2 tablespoons brown
    sugar or low-calorie
    sweetener suitable
    for baking

2 eggs
140 g (4 1/2 oz)
    unsweetened apple
    puree
1 cup (250 ml/8 fl oz)
    low-fat milk
olive oil spray

1 Sift the flour and baking powder into a bowl, stir in the sugar or sweetener and make a well in the centre. Whisk together the eggs, apple puree and milk. Pour into the well and whisk until smooth.
2 Lightly spray a fry pan with olive oil spray. Pour 1/4 cup (60 ml/2 fl oz) of the batter into the pan and cook over medium heat until bubbles appear on the surface. Turn and cook the other side. Keep warm while you cook the remaining batter.

per pancake (sugar) fat 1.7 g ▌ saturated fat 0.4 g ▌ protein 4.3 g ▌ carbohydrate 17.1 g ▌ fibre 2.5 g ▌ cholesterol 32 mg ▌ sodium 196 mg ▌ energy 442 kJ (106 Cal)

per pancake (sweetener) fat 1.7 g ▌ saturated fat 0.4 g ▌ protein 4.3 g ▌ carbohydrate 15.3 g ▌ fibre 2.5 g ▌ cholesterol 32 mg ▌ sodium 196 mg ▌ energy 414 kJ (99 Cal)

muesli   makes 7 cups

1 cup (65 g/2 oz) All-
    Bran® (processed
    wheat bran cereal)
3 cups (300 g/10 oz)
    rolled barley
1 cup (30 g/1 oz) wheat
    flakes
1/2 cup (50 g/1 2/3 oz)
    extruded rice bran
1 cup (75 g/2 1/2 oz)
    dried apples, chopped
1 cup (135 g/4 1/2 oz)
    dried apricots, chopped

2 tablespoons pepitas
2 tablespoons linseeds
    (flaxseeds)
2 tablespoons yellow
    box honey
1/3 cup (80 ml/2 2/3 fl oz)
    unsweetened low-GI
    apple juice
1 teaspoon ground
    cinnamon
1/2 teaspoon ground
    cardamom
1 teaspoon mixed spice

1 Preheat oven to 160°C (315°F/Gas 2–3). Line 2 baking trays with baking paper.
2 Put the All-Bran, barley, wheat flakes, rice bran, apples, apricots and seeds into a bowl. Mix to combine.
3 Put the honey, apple juice and spices into a pan. Bring to the boil, then pour over the dry ingredients and mix to combine. Spread on the prepared trays and bake for 30–35 minutes or until crisp and golden.

per cup fat 6 g ▌ saturated fat 0.9 g ▌ protein 8.9 g ▌ carbohydrate 64.7 g ▌ fibre 13.9 g ▌ cholesterol 0 mg ▌ sodium 65 mg ▌ energy 1471 kJ (351 Cal)

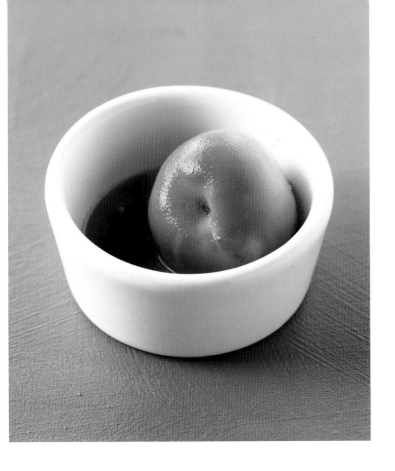

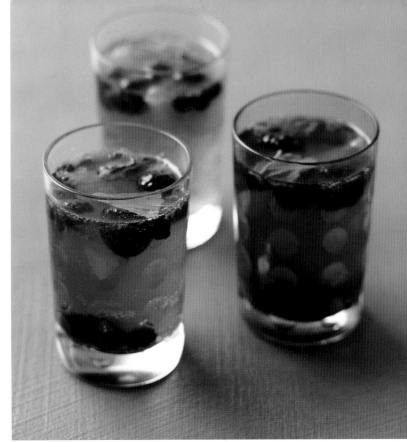

poached peaches serves 4

4 peaches
2 cups (500 ml/16 fl oz) unsweetened low-GI apple juice
1 cinnamon stick

3 star anise
4 cardamom pods, bruised
grated zest of 1 lemon
pinch of saffron threads

1 Cut a small cross in the top of each peach.
2 Put the apple juice, cinnamon stick, star anise, cardamom pods, lemon zest and saffron into a pan. Bring to the boil, then reduce the heat to a simmer.
3 Add the peaches and simmer for 5–10 minutes or until soft. Cool slightly, then peel off the skin before serving.

per serve fat 0.2 g ▮ saturated fat 0 g ▮ protein 1.2 g ▮ carbohydrate 22.8 g ▮ fibre 2 g ▮ cholesterol 0 mg ▮ sodium 15 mg ▮ energy 433 kJ (103 Cal)

party punch makes 10 cups

3¹/₂ cups (875 ml/ 28 fl oz) sparkling grape juice
3¹/₂ cups (875 ml/ 28 fl oz) unsweetened sparkling apple juice
850 ml (27 fl oz) unsweetened pineapple juice

few splashes of Angostura bitters (optional)
2 cups (250 g/8 oz) ice cubes
200 g (6¹/₂ oz) fresh or frozen mixed berries
1 orange, segmented
¹/₂ cup (25 g/1 oz) torn fresh mint

1 Put the grape juice, apple juice and pineapple juice into a large jug and gently stir to combine. Add the bitters, to taste, and chill until ready to serve.
2 Add the ice cubes, berries, orange and mint. Serve immediately.

per cup fat 0.1 g ▮ saturated fat 0 g ▮ protein 1 g ▮ carbohydrate 32.6 g ▮ fibre 0.9 g ▮ cholesterol 0 mg ▮ sodium 14 mg ▮ energy 574 kJ (137 Cal)

▮ Enjoy in moderation as an occasional treat.

index

recipes **Jody Vassallo** and **Tracey Gordon**
designer **Annette Fitzgerald**
consultant dietitian **Dr Susanna Holt**

styling **Jody Vassallo**
photographer **Sue Ferris**
props stylist **Vanessa Austin**
food for photography **Tracey Gordon**

editor **Justine Harding**

I can't believe it is five years since I started writing the very first *Diabetes* HEALTH FOR LIFE™ cookbook; time goes so fast and it is amazing how quickly the series has grown, and we now have big ideas as well. So firstly I would like to thank you, the person holding this book, for without you Fortiori would not have been able to grow and prosper as we have. I feel blessed to be able to write recipes for people who need them and who I know are going to use them (go on, give it a go!).

I also am honoured to work with an amazingly talented and dedicated team of people whom I cherish. None of what I do would be possible without my remarkable partners Claire, Helen and Peter; the hard work they do behind the scenes is necessary for each book to see the light of day. Thanks to my editor, Justine Harding, who returned to us from the cocoon of motherhood to oversee this project; bless you. Thanks to Annette Fitzgerald, our designer, for getting it all together in the nick of time before her overseas sojourn – I love the cover. Sue Ferris, my photographer, thank you for being such a pleasure to work and hang out with, you have done such a gorgeous job with this one. Thanks to Tracey Gordon or is that Gordon Tracey, my talented mate in the kitchen who makes my life easier, funnier and full of up-to-the-moment gossip. Susanna Holt, our dedicated dietitian, thanks for your tireless effort on this one. I know it's a subject close to your heart and one that you know more about than anyone I have ever met. Thank you for taking so much care in making sure that all the nutritional information we provide is totally accurate. Vanessa Austin, thanks for the lovely props and great paints.

And finally, thanks to my friends and family for your love and support as I continue to do what means so much to me. Thank you for the words of encouragement, the yums and scrums and the constructive criticism. A special mention to Matt, Relle, Rhearn and Nath for taking such great care of Pridey on days when she couldn't hang out with us at the studio; thanks, guys, I sometimes think she likes your place more than ours. To my Pridey girl, thanks for keeping me sane on the long drives to Sydney from Byron.

I would like to dedicate this book to my beloved friend Pat Manning, who passed away while I was making this book. Mornings at Bilgola will not be the same without you, mate. Lucky was I to have seen that cheeky face as often as I did.

Styling Credits

Alex Liddy 1300 763 833 ▯ Bison (02) 6257 7255 www.bisonhome.com ▯ Bodum (02) 9389 1488 www.bodum.com.au ▯ Deborah Hutton Homewares ▯ Design Mode International (02) 9998 8200 ▯ Dinosaur Designs (02) 9698 3500 www.dinosaurdesigns.com.au ▯ Elevate Designs 0413 637 385 www.elevatedesign.com.au ▯ Evans and Taylor (03) 9863 1133 ▯ Francalia (02) 9948 4977 www.francalia.com.au ▯ Gempo 1800 443 366 www.gempoliving.com.au ▯ Husk (03) 9528 7411 www.husk.com.au ▯ Kifkaf (02) 9699 3499 www.kifkaf.com.au ▯ Maxwell & Williams (03) 9318 0466 www.maxwellwilliams.com.au ▯ Mud Australia (02) 9699 7600 www.mudaustralia.com ▯ Rapee (02) 9496 4511 www.rapee.com.au ▯ Riess Enamelware (02) 4872 2295 www.goldfishent.com ▯ Rhubarb (03) 9429 9600 www.rhubarb.net.au ▯ Robert Gordon Australia (03) 5941 3302 www.robertgordonaustralia.com ▯ Sheldon & Hammond (02) 9482 6666 ▯ Studio Imports (03) 9530 9070 ▯ Tomkin (02) 9319 2993 www.tomkin.com.au ▯ Appliances used in this book provided by Sunbeam Corporation Limited.

This edition published in 2008 by GRUB STREET , 4 Rainham Close, London SW11 6SS
email: food@grubstreet.co.uk   www.grubstreet.co.uk

ISBN 978-1-904943-44-0

Printed in India.

DISCLAIMER: The nutritional information listed under each recipe does not include the nutrient content of garnishes or any accompaniments or ingredients not listed in specific quantities in the ingredient list (with the exception of oil sprays, where an estimated quantity is used). The nutritional information for each recipe is an estimate only, and may vary depending on the brand of ingredients used, and due to natural biological variations in the composition of natural foods such as meat, fish, fruit and vegetables. The nutritional information was calculated by a qualified dietitian using FoodWorks® dietary analysis software (Version 3.02, Xyris Software Pty Ltd, Highgate Hill, Queensland, Australia) based on Australian food composition data with additional data from food manufacturers and the American Department of Agriculture. Where not specified, ingredients are analysed as average or medium. All recipes were analysed using 59 g eggs.

An approximate glycemic index (GI) rating is also listed under the nutrient information for each recipe to indicate whether the dish produces a low, medium or high blood glucose response. The GI categories (low, medium or high) listed for each recipe are estimates only and were calculated by an experienced dietitian using published GI values for each of the carbohydrate-containing ingredients in the recipe. If an ingredient didn't have a published GI value, the GI value of the most similar foodstuff was used as a substitute. For this reason, and the fact that food preparation and cooking methods can affect a food's GI value, it is possible that some of the recipes may produce a higher or lower blood glucose response than predicted from the estimated GI rating listed. Therefore, it would be beneficial for people with diabetes to monitor their own individual blood glucose responses to the recipes, in order to determine which ones produce the lowest blood glucose responses.

This book is intended to provide general information only regarding diabetes and is not intended to replace any medical advice given to you by a qualified health professional. The authors and publisher cannot be held responsible for any adverse effects resulting from the use or misuse of the recommendations in this book or the failure to obtain or take appropriate medical advice.

IMPORTANT: Those who might suffer particularly adverse effects from salmonella food poisoning (the elderly, pregnant women, young children and those with immune system problems) should consult their general practitioner about consuming raw or undercooked eggs.